Place of Compassion

The fascinating story of a mountain Hospital in Lesotho, in Southern Africa.

About the Author

Kenneth Luckman was born in 1935 in Birmingham where he qualified as a doctor in 1958.

In 1961 he agreed to lead a pioneer medical project in the remote Maloti Mountains of Basutoland (now Lesotho).

He spent seven years helping to establish Saint James' Hospital, Mantšonyane in the heart of the mountains, to serve the needy rural Basotho farmers of the scattered villages. The hospital now serves the whole central area of Lesotho with a network of outlying clinics bringing curative and preventative medical care close to the people.

'Place of Compassion', his first book, relates the unique experience and difficulties of establishing the project from the beginning and it includes a fully researched account of the subsequent work of those who have carried the work forward into the new Millennium. Now retired from medical practice, he continues an interest in complementary medicine and serves as an Anglican Reader in Bromsgrove, Worcestershire. A further book on African beliefs and customs is in hand.

This book is also published by AuthorsOnLine in electronic format, details of which may be obtained at: www.authorsonline.co.uk

Author's Note.

The word 'compassion' means 'suffering with' or 'sharing the suffering of' the needy.

This book, which has been incubating for thirty years, is a twentieth century story of a pioneer work of Christian compassion.

A hospital may be found 7000 feet up in the Maloti Mountains of the African Kingdom of Lesotho in Southern Africa: the former High Commission Territory of Basutoland which became self governing in 1966.

I was privileged to be initially involved in this work for seven years and have recently revisited the Mission Hospital of Saint James at Mantšonyane which is now in its 38th year of serving the Basotho of central Lesotho with much needed medical care.

The Society for the Propagation of the Gospel (SPG), which had sponsored the project, made a short film about the hospital in 1963 called 'Place of Compassion'. I offer this fuller updated account in the hope that it may be of general interest, as a thanksgiving for all who have supported the work and as an inspiration for continued support in the 21st century.

Acknowledgements

I am indebted to the following for help and support with the book:

Annual Reports of St. James' Hospital;
Dr. Pamela Lorimer for her encouragement and helpful proof reading;
The LDA for their Newsletters;
My wife, Hazel, for her diaries, typing and maps;
My daughters, Rachel and Sarah, for their computer skills;
The USPG for their Newsletters to supporters.
For the following who have provided special contributions:
Dr. Nicholas Cohen;
Dr. Richard D'Aeth;
Rosalind Sellars (née Ferguson);
Dr. Simone Jaarsma;
Dr. Brian and Mrs Siân King;
The Rt. Reverend Desmond M. Tutu for the Foreword.

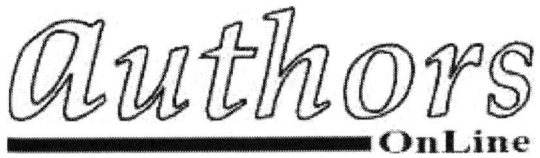

Place of Compassion

By

Dr Kenneth E Luckman

In memory of

John Arthur Arrowsmith Maund BA, MC, CBE
1909-1998
First Bishop of Lesotho

and

Petrose Lekolomi
1880-1963
A Basotho Chief

An AuthorsOnLine Book

Published by Authors OnLine Ltd 2001

Copyright © Authors OnLine Ltd

Text Copyright © Kenneth E Luckman

The front cover design of this book is produced by
Authors OnLine Ltd ©
Front cover photograph Kenneth Luckman ©
Rear cover portrait photograph is reproduced by kind permission of
Bailey's Studio, Bromsgrove, Worcestershire, England ©

The moral right of the author has been asserted.

All rights reserved. No part of this publication may be reproduced, stored in a retrieval system, or transmitted in any form or by any means, electronic, mechanical, photocopy, recording or otherwise, without prior written permission of the copyright owner. Nor can it be circulated in any form of binding or cover other than that in which it is published and without similar condition including this condition being imposed on a subsequent purchaser.

Printed and bound by Antony Rowe Limited, Eastbourne.

ISBN 0 7552 0028 4

Authors OnLine Ltd
15-17 Maidenhead Street
Hertford SG14 1DW
England

Visit us online at www.authorsonline.co.uk

Foreword
By The Rt Revd Desmond M Tutu,
former Archbishop of Capetown and second Bishop of Lesotho.

Missionaries have sometimes not had a good press. This unfortunate state of affairs has been occasioned by the fact that they were in times past frequently part of a triad that was the harbinger for colonial expansion and hegemony. I refer to the triad of missionary, trader and soldier. Many have believed that the missionary came to scout out the lie of the land and to soften up the natives for the advent of the trader and the militia who invariably staked out claims for the colonial power back in Europe. The cool ambivalence towards the missionary was captured in the oft told observation by a convert; 'When they (the missionaries) came, we had the land and they had the bible. Then they said, "Let us pray", and we duly shut our eyes; when we opened them, they had the land and we had the bible.'

There may be more than a modicum of truth in those tart remarks. But we can attest that there is another side of the story, a glorious side, one that can be told with exultant thanksgiving, especially here in southern Africa. Successive oppressive regimes in South Africa were not really too interested in the welfare of the indigenous majority of the population. Almost every African leader of any consequence in South Africa would testify that had it not been for the missionaries and the churches they would have had no education to speak of. Missionaries and the churches founded most of the major educational institutions in South Africa, which catered for blacks. The same would hold true for the provision of health services Those, that were sponsored by government were woefully inadequate in number and competence. So we could say that many of us would not have been alive today and many would not have been educated had it not been for the courage, altruism and dedication of some quite extraordinary people. These missionaries who left the comfort of their home countries to face the challenges of exotic lands and their people because of their dedication to the Lord who said, 'Go, make disciples of all people.'

Mantšonyane is the heart-warming story of the founding of one of these splendid health establishments founded by a dedicated band of outstanding people. The citizens of the Mountain Kingdom of Lesotho are deeply indebted to Dr Luckman and his colleagues.

As a former bishop of the diocese of Lesotho I can only try inadequately to say, '*Rea leboha, Ntate*'. We thank you, Father.'

Desmond M Tutu, Archbishop Emeritus   July 2001

Abbreviations Used In This Work

ACL	Anglican Church of Lesotho
AIDS	Acquired Immune Deficiency Syndrome
CEBEMO	Stichtung Nederland Lesotho
CEV	Contemporary English Version of the Bible
CHN	Community of the Holy Name, UK
CHAL	Church Hospitals' Association of Lesotho
EZE	Evangelische Zentrallstall fur Entwicklung-schilfe
DOG	Dienst over Grenzen
FWD	Four Wheel Drive
HC	Health Centre
HSA	Health Service Area
LEC	Lesotho Evangelical Church
LFDS	Lesotho Flying Doctor Service
LDA	Lesotho Diocesan Association, UK
MAF	Missionary Aviation Fellowship
NLT	New Living Translation of the Bible
PEMS	Paris Evangelical Missionary Society
PHAL	Private Hospitals' Association of Lesotho
PHC	Primary Health Care
SPB	Society of the Precious Blood, UK
SPG	Society for the Propagation of the Gospel, UK
SSM	Society of the Sacred Mission, UK
STD	Sexually Transmitted Disease
TNA	Trained Nursing Assistant
TBA	Traditional Birth Attendant
UFC	Under- Five Clinic
USPG	United Society for the Propagation of the Gospel, UK (an amalgamation of SPG and the Universities Mission to Central Africa)
VHP	Village Health Post
VHW	Village Health Worker

Lesotho: its position in Southern Africa

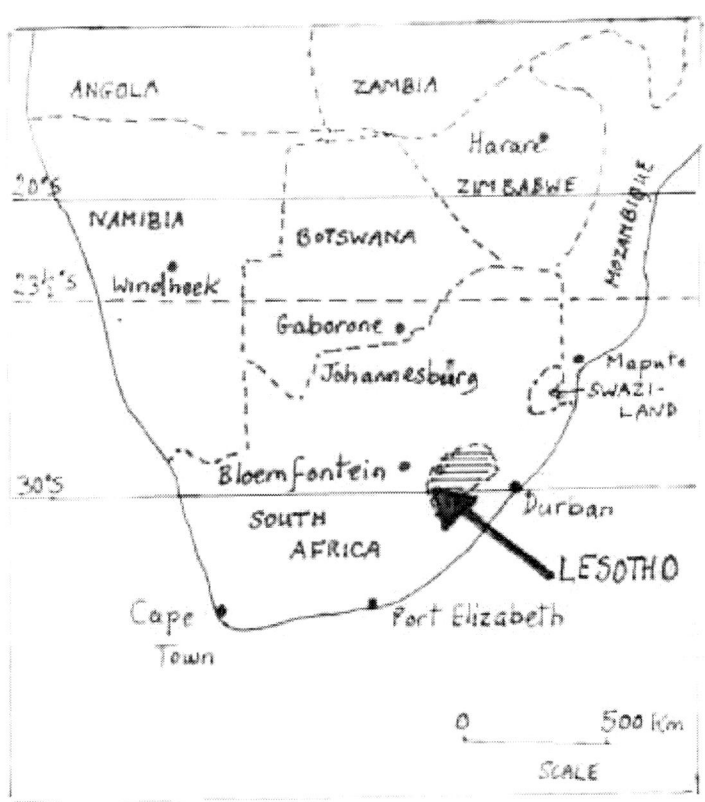

The Position of Lesotho in Southern Africa

Mantšonyane Health Service Area in Lesotho

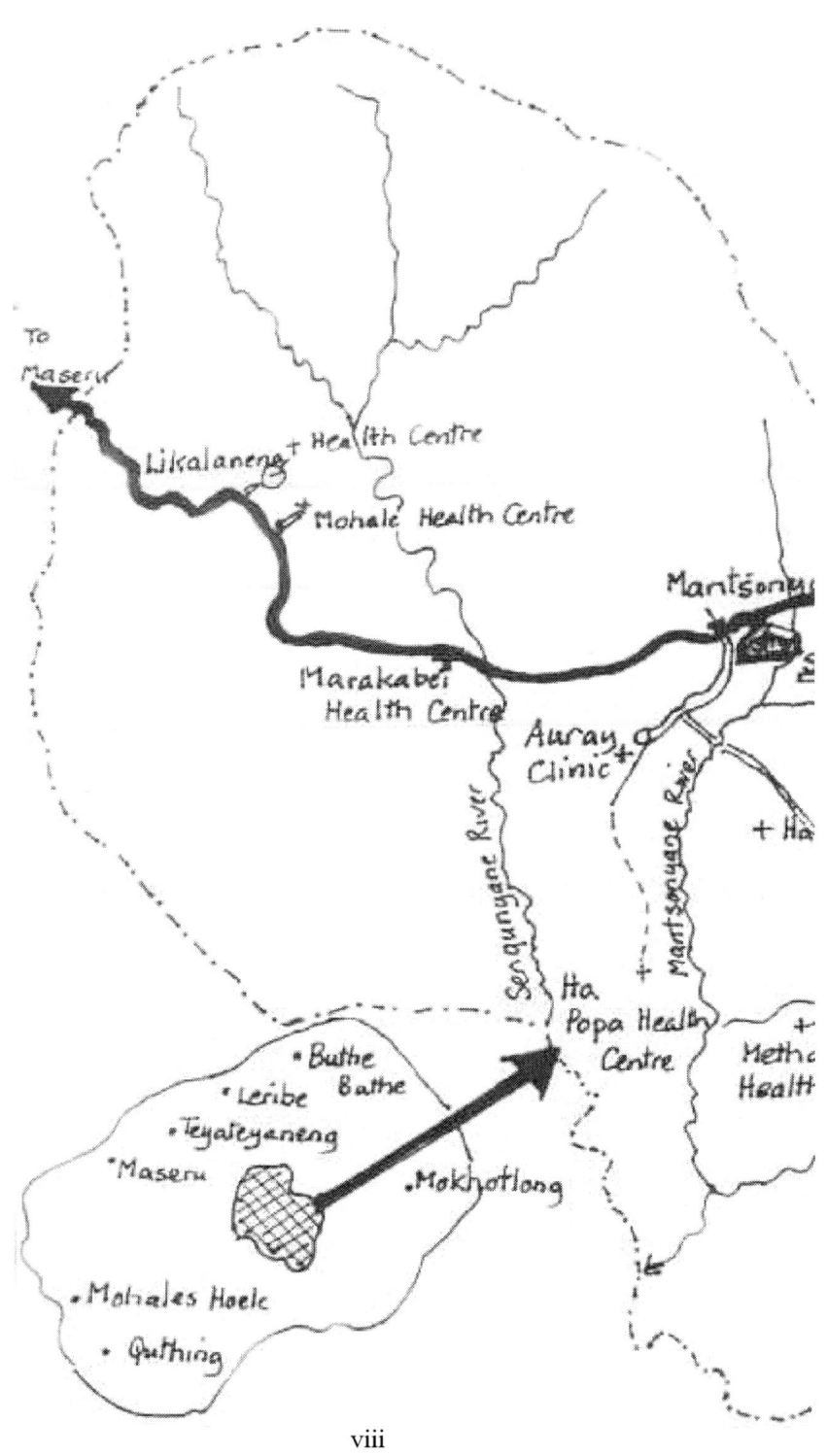

Mantšonyane Health Service Area in Lesotho

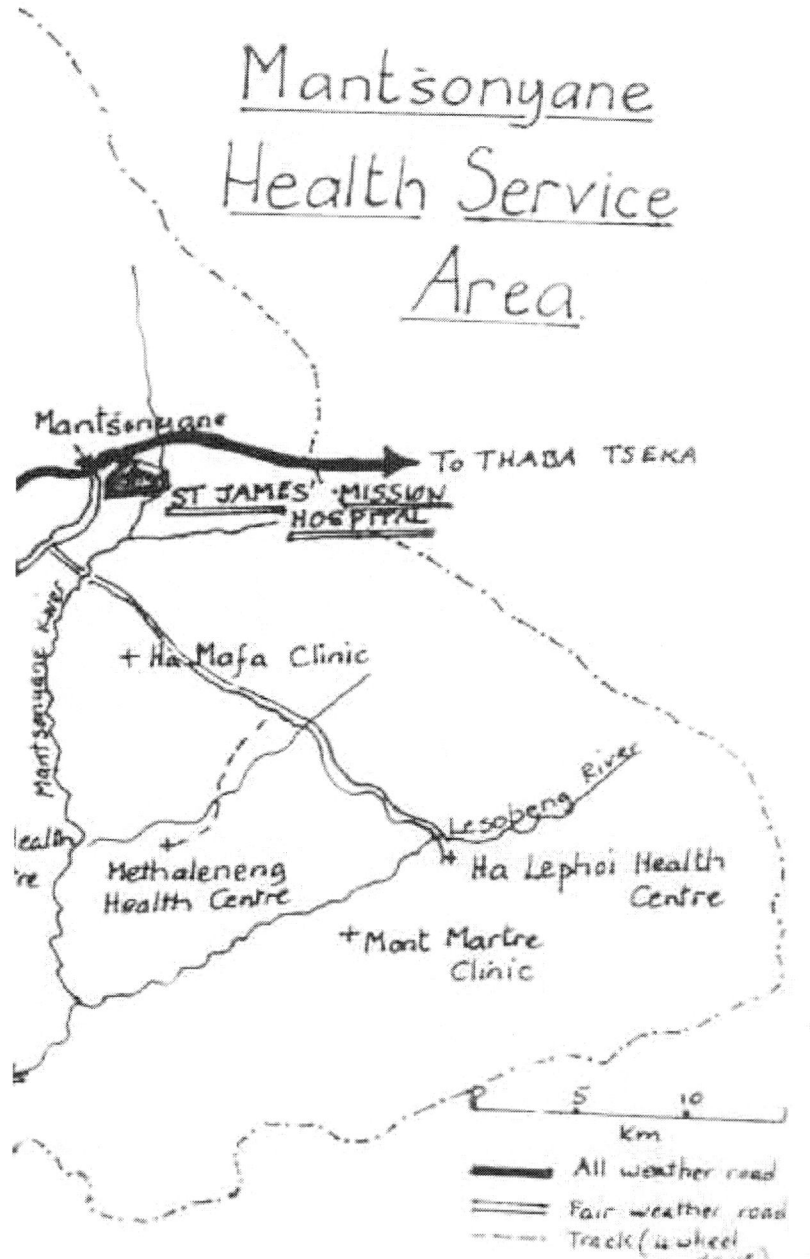

The opening of St James Hospital

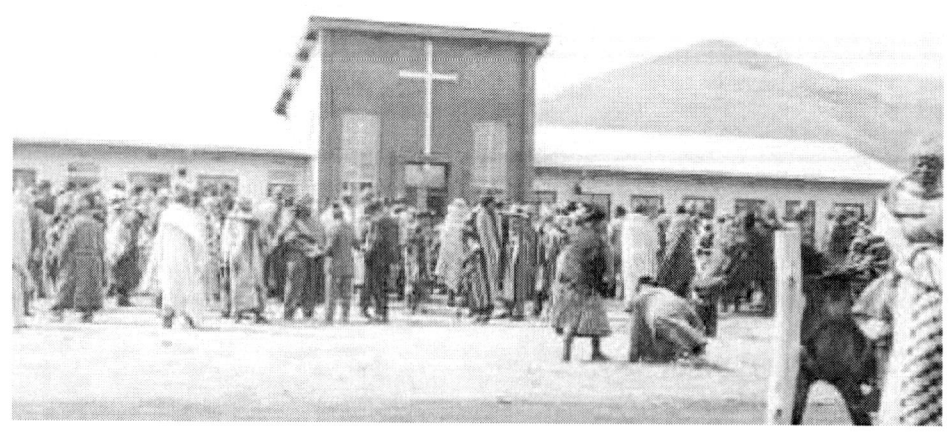

CONTENTS

PART I: CHAPTERS 1-4

1	How it all began.	1
2	The early days.	9
3	The first phase of building.	16
4	The second phase of building.	28

PART II: CHAPTERS 5-13

5	Unexpected help.	40
6	Consolidation of confidence.	49
7	Help from South Africa.	60
8	Difficult times.	67
9	Rescue from the Netherlands.	70
10	Sustained help from the Netherlands.	75
11	Towards the Millennium.	87
12	The Primary Health Care Programme.	101
13	Past, present and future	113

SESOTHO-ENGLISH VOCABULARY	122
USEFUL ADDRESSES	122

St. James Hospital Today

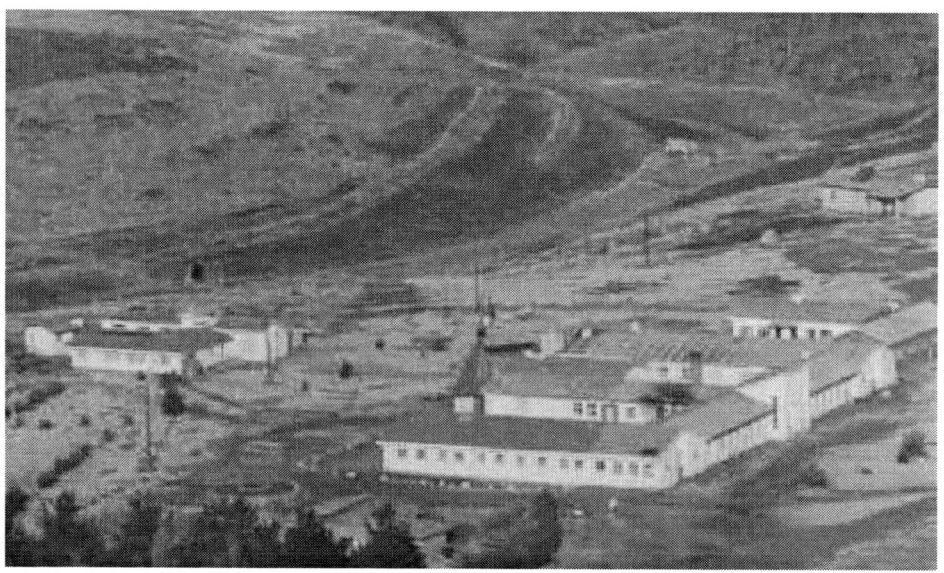

PART ONE.

Chapter 1: HOW IT ALL BEGAN.

'I look up to the mountains-does my help come from there?'
(Ps 121.1 NLT).

The ubiquitous fascination of the human race for mountains is well known from antiquity. The great bare mass of volcanic rock known as the Maloti Mountains, 6,000 to 11,000 feet above sea level, constitutes the Eastern two thirds of Lesotho, which is a dissected plateau 200 million years old.
The highest point of Southern Africa, Thaba Ntlenyana is 11,425 feet above sea level, in the eastern Drakensberg mountain range bordering on Natal.
The Basotho people were formed from the different clans of the Sotho-Tswana racial group. They migrated to Tafelkop now in the Free State, west of the present Lesotho, in the latter part of the 18th century. Originally they came from what is now Botswana, formerly known as Bechuanaland, and before that probably from North-East Africa.
By 1830 Moshoeshoe the Great had welded scattered clans into one nation. By 1851 the Basotho had been expelled from the fertile lands of the Orange Free State by Dutch farmers who pushed them back across the Caledon River into the less fertile lands of what is now the lowlands of Lesotho.
In 1868 Moshoeshoe asked for protection by Queen Victoria to avoid being swallowed up into what was to become the Union of South Africa. This British High Commission territory of 11,716 square miles thus became an enclave completely surrounded by the present Republic of South Africa. In the late 19th and early 20th century many Basotho gradually migrated from the lowlands into the foothills and mountains, owing to overcrowding and lack of land for grazing and cultivation. The areas to which they moved were virtually treeless and relatively infertile grasslands with little good grazing for their animals. Mantšonyane (Little Black River) was just such an area in the central Maloti mountains and Ha Chooko was a typical medium sized village on the East side of the Mantšonyane River which was a tributary of the Orange river (Senqu).
The Anglican Church began work in the lowlands in 1876. Sometime after the Spanish Influenza Epidemic (Mokakalane) of 1918 a church and later a school were established at Ha Chooko with a resident Mosotho (singular of Basotho) catechist in charge. At Christmas and Easter a priest would ride more than 50 miles from Saint Mark's church, Masapong, Ha Theko, in the lowlands to celebrate mass for the congregation (In Sesotho 'Missa' is the commonly used title for the service of the Eucharist or Holy Communion in the Anglican and Roman Catholic Churches.)

At this time, Basutoland was part of the Diocese of Bloemfontein in the Orange Free State and was cared for by an assistant bishop of the diocese and it was not until 1950 that Basutoland became a separate diocese with its own bishop. John Maund was chosen by Archbishop Clayton of Capetown to be the first Bishop of Basutoland and from the first he signed himself: '+John Lesotho', thus anticipating the reversion of the anglicised 'Basutoland' to 'Lesotho', the original African name of the country, adopted officially after self-government. This was typical of Bishop Maund's approach to the Basotho people with whom he was to identify closely and serve so unstintingly for the next 25 years. Bishop Maund lost no time in getting to know his new diocese. In 1951, the year following his consecration, he visited Ha Chooko village at Mantšonyane on horseback – the Mountain Road was still 12 miles away at Ha Marakabei on the far side of the Senqunyane river. On this first visit the bishop called on the headman of Ha Chooko, Petrose Lekolomi who was then 71 years of age, being born at the time of the Gun War (Ntoa ea Lithunya) in 1880.

Morena (Chief) Chooko pleaded with the bishop to send a resident priest for his village and also to find a doctor to serve the needy people of the area. Bishop Maund promised the old chief that he would do what he could about both these requests. On the 16th October 1952, Father Phillip Stroud, of the 'Society of the Sacred Mission', (S S M), was sent by the bishop to take up residence at Ha Chooko and became the first Rector of St James' parish, Mantšonyane to serve a network of outstations throughout the central Maloti area.

In the following year of 1953 I was 18 years of age and was about to commence medical training at the Medical School of Birmingham University. That summer I attended a Summer School organised by the SPG at Broadstairs in Kent. During that week I learned a great deal about the world-church and its needs. Whilst listening to an organ recital a powerful and unexpected thought came into my mind: 'You are to work as a doctor in the Third World!' This was a bolt from the blue, as I had no idea what I wanted to do with my life. I was just about to start medical studies and had doubts as to whether I would survive the course. However, the idea of overseas service just didn't go away.

About half way through the medical course, Doctor Anthony Barker returned to his 'Alma Mater' and spoke to us about his work at Nqutu in Zululand – very much a pioneer medical mission run together with his wife Maggie, during the last decade or so. There was no longer any real doubt in my mind about the sort of work I was being called to do.

After qualification as a doctor in 1958 I worked at Selly Oak Hospital, Birmingham and Coventry and Warwickshire Hospital, Coventry. I was just completing an obstetric post at Bromsgrove General Hospital when I received a letter from Father Paul Hume SSM, the Director of the Society of the Sacred Mission, at Kelham in Nottinghamshire. The letter said: 'We are looking for a doctor to work in a pioneer medical project in the mountains of Basutoland' – another bolt from the blue!

I had never heard of Father Hume or the religious community of which he was superior. I knew extremely little about Basutoland, apart from the issue of stamps commemorating the Royal Visit there in 1947 – It was somewhere in Africa! A hasty recourse to an ancient encyclopaedia told me that it was a tiny mountain Kingdom, well South of the equator, where I thought I might survive! In an act of faith - some would say a fit of sheer madness, I agreed to accept the job, if I were thought to be suitable. The Archbishop's Board gave their approval and the SPG agreed to sponsor me.

Arrangements were soon underfoot for a preparatory term at the House of the Sacred Mission, the mother-house of the Kelham Fathers and their theological college in Nottinghamshire. This proved a welcome breathing space after 8 years of medical study and hospital practice. I was able to do some useful anthropological and theological study and began to learn the Sesotho language with Isaac Dhlamini, a delightful African lay novice of the Society. It was also useful to be able to get to know some of the Kelham Fathers who had worked in Basutoland for many years. Their experience was invaluable and encouraging.

Knowing that we would be faced with Tuberculosis as a major problem I was glad to work in a Chest Clinic in Newark nearby. Most of all I learned something about living in a close Christian community of very varied people and the value of a balanced life of prayer, work and leisure.

A letter from Bishop Maund did not minimise the toughness of the initial work in starting the project from scratch and in living in quite primitive conditions. So, at the age of 26 on the 26th of January 1961 I boarded the Royal Mail Steamer 'Caernarvon Castle' for the 14-day cruise from Southampton to Capetown. The sadness of leaving home, family and friends was tempered by the beginning of an exciting adventure.

By this time I had been joined by two colleagues. Arnold Skelton, a rotund 37 year-old Liverpudlian, was a State Registered Nurse and accomplished opera singer with many other practical abilities. Gerald Garroway from Buckinghamshire was 24 and a builder who already had experience in South West Africa. We were faced with a press conference on-board ship before sailing. This resulted in a photograph of the three of us, which made the back page of the Church Times with a catchy journalistic caption 'Three men go up a mountain to build a hospital!'

The cruise was helpful in getting to know each other as we shared an outer cabin. We also had opportunity of meeting a number of seasoned missionaries from various parts of Africa and a few newer recruits like ourselves.

Major Kirby and his wife of the Salvation Army, returning to Rhodesia (later Zimbabwe) impressed us greatly with a very practical approach to mission. In an ecumenical bible study Major Kirby pointed out that when Jesus sent his disciples for the ass and colt he had made all the necessary preparations beforehand – and this he always did! This struck a chord with us as we started out on our journey of faith together.

On another occasion John Carter, designated for a chaplaincy at Cape Town University said: 'Christians must expect to suffer, who knows what lies ahead of us in Africa?'.During our voyage we had plenty of time to discuss tentative plans. There was a lot of hard thinking and praying to be done as we contemplated our daunting task ahead. Only Arnold was brave enough to agree with Major Kirby to give a testimony about his vocation, which had arisen out of his membership of the Nurse' Christian Fellowship.

After two weeks of deck games, lager and lime and too much food, provided by the Union Castle line, we were excited to reach Cape Town on February 9th at dawn. Table Mountain was shrouded with a blanket of mist and we saw the brown earth of Africa for the first time. We lost no time in boarding the so-called 'Orange Express' train for Durban in Natal. We spent three days and two nights chugging through the dusty Karoo up to the Orange Free State, stopping leisurely at numerous small *dorps* (small rural towns) and being interrogated by friendly South Africans. We skirted around Basutoland, passed into the more wooded country of Natal to Durban on the coast. We were met at Durban by Dr. John and Mrs. Clare Currie who slewed us through red-mudded roads and heavy rain in a Volkswagen Beetle to arrive at their hospital of St. Mary, KwaMagwaza, after dark in a humid heat. We soon fell asleep in spite of the deafening sound of crickets, after a 17-day journey with so much to take in.

We awoke next morning to see the full beauty of the wooded hills of Zululand (now KwaZulu) and attended Zulu Mass in the hospital chapel – we were enthralled with the lusty Zulu singing. Arnold was put in charge of the male ward and Gerry set to work with Mr. Pawley the maintenance man while I did a round of the hospital with John Currie – we finished the morning round at 3pm!

Arnold and I were to spend 7 weeks at St. Mary's. We learned very much about African medicine and nursing in this time, although Amoebic Dysentery and Bilharzia were unknown the other side of the Drakensberg mountains, in our final destination of Basutoland. Whilst at KwaMagwaza I learned to extract teeth and performed my first extraction on the 14th February, the first day of Decimal currency in South Africa – it came out in one piece, Alleluia! My first visit to an out-station clinic was to Springfield. All went well until we heard a tremendous commotion outside. The nurse with me screamed 'there's a snake outside' and promptly jumped up on the examination couch. Meanwhile I slammed the door firmly shut and prayed hard. Shortly the panic outside subsided and I cautiously opened the door and peered out to find a very small black snake whose life had been quickly terminated by the Zulu men standing round it in triumph.

The following week we visited the famous Charles Johnson Hospital at Nqutu and spent a few hours with Doctors Anthony and Maggie Barker who had visited my Medical School some six years previously. They went to Zululand in 1945 and had built up their hospital from almost nothing in fifteen years. At Nqutu we met Doctor Ted Nottidge who had been up to Mantšonyane in the previous year to make an initial survey of the possibility of building a Hospital there.

According to Ted, the area we would be expected to cover contained 20 to 25,000 Basotho living in scattered villages within a radius of about 50 miles. The Mountain Road was a dirt road built with a grant from the UK. Transport costs would be high but Murray and Neal Yeats, the owners of the trading store, had already promised help for taking up hospital needs and there was a radio transmitter at the store, which we would be welcome to use for contact with Maseru, the capital. A doctor from the Orange Free State had been well patronised on his visits to the local store. There was probably enough work for 7 doctors! It was too late for second thoughts now! An initial legacy for £15,000 had been left by a Miss Purser of Sidcup, Kent, specifically for medical missionary work and SPG had assigned this to our project. We were pleased to learn that the Mine Recruitment organisation had agreed to provide a further £10,000 when the building was underway.

Ted Nottidge had recommended a small unit at first with outlying village clinics staffed by Basotho Nurses. He suggested small casualty and maternity units as the first priority. He also thought that domiciliary work would be important in building up confidence and also as an effective measure towards health education. All this gave us much food for thought.

Back at St Mary's we had to take full charge of the hospital with its 200 beds while John and Clare took a much needed holiday. We had to learn how to take x-rays and develop them. We managed to cope with all the varied problems for the two weeks on our own – a foretaste of things to come.

By this stage Gerry was champing at the bit to go to Basutoland. This was agreed with Bishop Maund so that he might make some basic temporary domestic arrangements at Ha Chooko whilst living at St James' Mission.

In early April we left KwaMagwaza and Clare drove us to Durban where we boarded the train to Modderport in the Orange Free State. Brother Aidan SSM met us off the train and we spent three weeks at the SSM Priory of St. Augustine. On arrival Bishop Maund was waiting to meet us. We took to him immediately as he proved such a friendly down-to-earth person with a great sense of humour. We came to know him as Bishop John, a wise counsellor over the years – kind, thoughtful and holy in the best sense of the word. Bishop John was just as much at home scrambling along a mountain track in faded blue jeans and a cowboy hat, as when officiating in cope and mitre at a confirmation. Of all the bishops in the Anglican Communion not one had more justification for wearing gaiters, as he spent many weeks a year in the saddle visiting his scattered flock. He had been 11 years running the diocese on a shoe string and had accomplished a great deal in his close pastoral contacts with the Basotho, founding new churches and schools and now, to his great delight, the first hospital. While he spoke with us on the stoep (verandah) at Modderport Priory his enthusiasm rather ran away with him as he sketched a plan of the proposed hospital site on the mud smeared wall of the priory, much to the disgust of Father Prior who muttered something about episcopal desecration!

The Bishop explained to us that we were to experience the very worst climatic conditions on our arrival as winter was approaching and we were likely to have snow and possibly be cut off from Maseru for some periods of time. We gazed together across the flat Free State farmland to the distant Maloti Mountains which could just be seen enveloped in a blue haze – our future home for some years to come.

Arnold and I were able to do some further language study. What a strange sight it must have been to see two grown men sitting in the back row of the infants' class learning to count in Sesotho and imitate the pronunciation of a new, beautiful but strange language.

During the next week or two we took our very first lessons in horse riding down at Modderport Farm under the watchful eye of Dick Vogts, the Farm Manager. We were never thrown off but were pretty scared when the horses started to canter with us astride with no saddle or stirrups!

During our stay at Modderport the whole community of SSM Fathers arrived for their Easter Retreat. The last to arrive were Father Clement and Father Donald with whom we would be working at Chooko's. There was a very marked contrast of personalities which was typical of the community as a whole. Father Clement was a clever linguist and something of a scholar and came from a Norfolk family. Father Donald was a former sheep farmer from South Australia – a quiet man of great practical ability in such matters as putting on a church roof and could he ride a horse!

In parting Bishop John had suggested we might buy a second hand Austin Gypsie which we could run into the ground during the initial building work. Unfortunately Dick Vogts didn't think it would survive in the Maloti. In fact a trial of the vehicle only just managed to get us to Maseru for the second meeting of the new hospital board!

This first venture into the capital city of Basutoland was a revelation. In those days Maseru was like a Wild West town together with horse hitching posts and clouds of dust. The buildings were of Colonial type with trading stores and a few imposing new buildings such as the Queen Elizabeth Hospital, Law Court and Legislative Council buildings. We were graciously entertained by a South African businessman and his wife, Horace and Winifred Coaker. Their home on the outskirts of the town was called 'Pono e ntle' (Beautiful Sight). It was to become a second home to us three on our occasional trips down from the mountains and we were always welcome.

On the 1st of May we moved from Modderport to 'Pono e ntle' for nearly three weeks and both gained experience working at the QEII Government Hospital – I was in the Out Patients department and Arnold in the wards.

On the 17th May Winnie Coaker took us up to the end of the Mountain Road for the first time for a day visit. The trip of nearly 80 miles took 6 hours before we reached the future hospital site. Over the last 10 miles of road the hairpin bends were so numerous I never succeeded in counting them during my 7 years of using the road.

When we first saw the bare plateau surrounded by towering mountains we were told that our faces were completely expressionless. We had come up through a dangerous pass called 'Molimo Nthuse' which meant 'God Help Me'. That indeed was our sentiment as we silently contemplated the mass of rock covered with little grass on which we were to establish the hospital. Gerry had reacted similarly three months before on his arrival. His prayer was "My God…………Amen" – with a thousand thoughts between 'My God' and "Amen!". We were going to need God's help without a doubt!

Father Donald met us with horses from Ha Chooko, half a mile across the Mantšonyane Gorge. The horses took us reluctantly down the grassy slope to the river, which was only ankle deep with water. There was a square flat rock in the river and we were advised never to attempt to cross if this rock were covered with water. We then clambered up a steep rocky path to St James' Mission in the centre of Ha Chooko village which was to be our temporary home in less than three weeks. We were met at the mission by Father Clement in fur hat and cape – winter had just begun!

We were pleased with the progress Gerry had made in converting thatched mud and stone round huts (*rondavels*) into more habitable dwellings. We had lunch with the Fathers and then attended Benediction in the new Church of St James built about 5 years before by Father Clement. We retraced our way back to Maseru getting back just before dark. It was a full day. What had we landed ourselves into?

On the following day we ordered basic medical supplies from Bloemfontein in the Orange Free State and collected Penicillin, Streptomycin and Anti-TB drugs from the government stores, which were provided for Tuberculosis and Venereal Diseases. The next day we learned that the hospital was to be called 'St James English Church Mission Hospital'. This was rather too much of a mouthful for me. I agreed with the patronage of St James' following the dedication of our Pro-Cathedral in Maseru. I thought this was enough indication of who would be responsible for the new hospital and preferred to drop the 'English Church' bit as unnecessary and a bit outdated. Eventually it was accepted that we be 'St James' Mission Hospital'.

Our last 10 days in the lowlands were spent at Morija, about 28 miles from Maseru where we spent a very useful time with Dr. Ted Germond at the Scott Hospital run by the French Protestant Church. Ted was a third generation missionary – his great grandfather had been a member of the second group of missionaries sent by the Paris Evangelical Missionary Society in the 19th Century. His out patients' clinics seemed to go all day with a wealth of clinical cases including the first patient I had ever seen with Diphtheria.

From Morija we visited Masite and visited the Sisters of the 'Society of the Precious Blood', (SPB), from Burnham who had been praying for us for a long time. We returned to Masite for our last days before going up to Mantšonyane to stay. The Archdeacon, Father Maurice James promised to get some roomy saddle-bags made for us by one of his churchwardens.

Chapter 2. THE EARLY DAYS

'My help will come from the Lord who created the heavens and the earth.'
(Ps 121.2 CEV)

On 1st June 1961, after Corpus Christi Mass at St James' Pro-Cathedral in Maseru, Arnold and I set out in a new Land Rover laden with our personal possessions and basic medical supplies. At last we were on the last lap before rejoining our colleague Gerry at Ha Chooko. We completed the journey to Mantšonyane in about 4 hours. After unloading at the hospital site we were met by Aaron Tsoako with the mission mule, a beast of 20 years of age who knew every track in the parish. We had been warned by the Bishop never to stand behind this mule who had in the past kicked him savagely. The mule carried most of our belongings. Bulk supplies were already being stored at the Trading Store of Collier and Yates at the end of the Mountain Road proper and ¼ of a mile from the 'hospital site'. There was one large heavy case filled with books that even the mule couldn't manage. We were standing wondering how on earth to transport this weighty object, when one of the ladies from the village with one sweep placed it on her head and tripped off happily down the valley. We had learned our first lesson: Basotho women were resourceful, strong and industrious. We negotiated the ascent to Ha Chooko ourselves on horseback arriving in time for lunch, in our new home at last.

Our accommodation consisted of three traditional round huts built of local stone (rondavels) with conical thatched roofs, mud and cattle dung smeared on the walls and floors. Gerry had been very busy putting in extra windows, substantial doors, fitted shelves and cupboards. He also had acquired basic furniture of beds, tables and chairs, together with household necessities. The largest rondavel was to be mine with the dubious privilege of serving as a common room and dining room as well.

Through the stable-type door of my rondavel I could see St James' cement block church up the hill as well as the stone built school which had originally served as a church. Just behind my residence was a rectangular cement block building with a corrugated iron roof which had been built by Father Clement, about five years before to serve as a dispensary, staffed for a time by a nurse, Miss Dora Pennington. Previous to her a male nurse, Fred Warren, had also worked at Ha Chooko for a short time in 1954.

The old dispensary had been renovated by Gerry and he had converted part of it into a kitchen with a cooker run from gas cylinders, the rest to serve as a temporary clinic so that we could start seeing patients on the spot, straightaway. A barbed wire fence had been erected to enclose the dispensary grounds from stray animals. We were right in the centre of the village, near to the spring where all water had to be fetched by hand. The two parts of the village, divided by a stream, were on either side of us. We had to go up to the mission to share their primitive toilet. We washed in basins on stands using hot water stored in thermos flasks in piece-meal fashion, sometimes using the antiquated shower at the mission built by the first priest, Phillip Stroud eight years previously.

This was how we lived for our first nine months in the midst of a friendly Basotho community who accepted us as a matter of course and made us feel at home. During those first few months we got to know the people and made strenuous efforts to improve our Sesotho; their beautiful language was a vital challenge to us. I spent many sunsets just sitting by the village spring and listening to the women and children chattering as they came to draw water. The older women spoke more slowly and were easier to follow while the children were quite uninhibited in correcting our faltering attempts to speak with them. The small children's language was at first just what we needed. Later on it was the grandmothers and grandfathers who taught me most. No wonder I was later told I spoke like the much-respected older generation and also with a mountain accent which tended to drawl the vowels. The Sesotho I learned in the village together with an old grammar book written by a French Protestant missionary, partly explained how amused lowlanders were to hear such old fashioned language which was I think a purer form of the language, before it had been influenced from outside. Although I never attained the fluency of an expert, I more than got by with every day matters and medical work, within a year, due to actually living in the village for three quarters of that time.

While Arnold and Gerry went flat out working on the building site I had more time to devote to language study before the medical work escalated. Visiting people at home with a guide was time consuming but also very helpful: not only linguistically but also in learning exactly how people lived; which was often an important factor in their health problems. We employed a young Roman Catholic Mosotho, Martin Moejane, as an interpreter fairly early on and he was a great help to us in those early months. It was good, that gradually I was able to cope without an interpreter after the first few months – apart from delicate and intricate problems and even then it was not always easy to find a really reliable interpreter. I soon realised that to be fairly fluent in two languages does not mean that one will necessarily interpret well. I found many Basotho so polite that they would say what they thought you *should say*, rather than what you actually *said*. Also, to translate idiomatically is a skill not easily acquired. It was a joy when I could follow a Sesotho church service without difficulty and a little later to take a more vocal part. After 6 months I was able to take prayers in Sesotho when the Fathers were away.

On our first morning at Ha Chooko our very first out patient arrived with raging toothache and we had to hastily unpack one of our bags to find the dental forceps. The painless extraction of a tooth was a great confidence builder. Father Clement, like many priests could perform this procedure but without a local anaesthetic!

On our third day Father Donald took me up the village to pay my respect to the local headman, Petrose Lekolomi, whom Bishop John had first visited 10 years before. He was now 81 years old. Morena Chooko could just be made out as we entered his smoke filled rondavel. He was a wizened figure with droopy eyelids and shaven head, seated on a mud floor. After the usual greetings were exchanged, Father Donald said: 'This is 'Ntate Ngaka' ("Mr. Doctor")'. The old chief expressed his delight at our arrival and wished to know how soon we would be starting work. He also assured us he would help if we had any problems with his people in the village – in fact we never did. He then went on to insist on being examined there and then for his aches and pains. I obliged and could find little wrong with the chief apart from muscular rheumatism and 'Anno Domini'. He then made a request I was to hear very many times: 'Ke batla ente' (I want an injection). I took my professional reputation in my hands and made it clear that I didn't think he needed an injection but would send him a bottle of medicine to ease his aches and pains. The universal desire of the Basotho for injections and their belief that they could cure anything had arisen from the common practice of early government doctors in the lowlands of giving everybody an injection of Vitamin B for malnutrition, which no doubt many people had suffered from.

After visiting the chief we then called on our first real medical visit to see a lady with a septic bursitis of her knee (infected Housemaid's Knee). She did require an injection of Penicillin and was treated with a whole course of injections over the next week.

Morena (Chief) Chooko was actually only a minor headman in his own village of about 600 people and came under the local chief, Toka Mojela on whose land we were to build the hospital. Morena Toka was quite an educated man but had fallen victim to the 'white man's beer' of Brandy and was in a fairly advanced state of chronic alcoholism when I first met him. In fact I only saw him in a remotely sober condition on one or two occasions during my whole time at Mantšonyane. When chief Toka visited the hospital site to fix the boundary fence he was bleary eyed and walked with a stagger and would have given us anything we wanted in exchange for a bottle of Brandy. However, I resolutely refused to fuel his alcohol addiction with bribes and said that we were there to build a hospital for his people and the least he could do was to provide us with sufficient land. When summoned to see him medically I never lost an opportunity of warning him that he was killing himself with alcohol; but he never headed this advice and died several years later on, still in middle age.

We soon settled in our temporary quarters which were heated by paraffin stoves on the very cold nights of our first winter. On one occasion I went to bed fully clothed, wearing a deer-stalker and hugging a hot water bottle. We used Tilley lamps fuelled also by paraffin. These gave a very good light although in the warmer months attracted a myriad of moths whose bodies had to be cleaned out of the glass globes weekly.

Before Arnold and I had arrived Gerry had set on a domestic staff for us of no less than four Basotho; which seemed to me a little in excess of our requirements. I began to appreciate the need when I started to train Adolphina Poone to do some cooking for us. She was a delightful person and very willing but slow to learn simple Western style cooking. She was a young widow with a most angelic face. Her husband, a Catechist, had been drowned in the Mantšonyane river trying to cross in full flood – a salutary warning to us. Adolphina's first lessons were a hoot, with a pocket dictionary in one hand and a simple cookery book in the other. The results were soon edible but rarely did she manage to cook potatoes long enough and her first attempts at tea making were not very successful. Poor Adolphina never quite managed to lay a table perfectly.

Early on Gerry asked her to bring in some bananas which he had brought up from Maseru. Gerry said 'Ak'u tlise banana' ('please bring in the bananas'). The look of bewilderment on her face as she shuffled out to the kitchen puzzled us. A few minutes later she returned but without any bananas. We repeated our request several times slowly. A hasty search of a pocket dictionary revealed no word for banana in Sesotho but, I recalled banana was the plural of 'ngoanana' that meant 'girl'! The mystery was solved. Adolphina thought that she was being asked to bring girls from the village. When I said Ak'u tlise 'tholoana e tsehla' (the yellow fruit), all the misunderstanding was resolved and Adolphina's face broke in to a toothy grin. The mountain Basotho had never seen bananas.

Adolphina was assisted by her sister-in-law, Augustina, who was responsible for washing and ironing thoroughly but in slow motion, and if she were left on her own for any length of time she would drift of into a pleasant slumber. Eventually, we removed the seat from the kitchen until the week's washing had been completed. This solved the problem.

The other two members of the domestic staff were men. Dyke was Augustina's husband and was a fine muscular man who had worked in the mines of South Africa, as so many able bodied men did at the time. They would send money home at regular intervals to support their families.

Dyke was not 'overbright' and used to fetch and carry goods from the trading store across the river. This work usually took at least two hours longer than expected and he always returned smelling unmistakably of 'Joala' (Sesotho beer). Augustina and Dyke produced an infant who arrived into this world in quite a hurry just before I arrived at their rondavel to conduct the delivery. Augustina was back at work in a few days. This was not unusual. Sometimes at harvest time a Mosotho woman would give birth in the fields and then carry on reaping the harvest! The baby would be wrapped in a blanket and carried round on the back. This mode of transport resulted in babies very rarely suffering from wind.

The other man, John, who worked for us was a very thin smart fellow with beady eyes and a quick guilty smile. He was employed to look after the three horses we had acquired. We named them after the three English counties from which the three of us had come, although as it worked out we hardly ever rode the horse bearing the name of our own particular county. Hence Gerry rode the beautiful red stallion called Warwick, Arnold rode the lovely Basotho pony called Buckingham who could be quite mischievous, which made the Basotho call him 'Baroa' (Bushmen). I rode the slightly larger Basotho pony called Lancaster. John cared for the horses well but eventually fell from grace when he started helping himself to horse feed for his own horse. We found eventually that Dyke could in fact manage the horses and transport and he had less time to imbibe the local brew. We were never able to manage with only one lady.

A task which Adolphina really liked was re-smearing the rondavel floors with mud and cattle dung which left an unpleasant odour for days afterwards. Consequently, we usually tried to curb Adolphina's enthusiasm and arrange for her to do this job while the occupant was away for a few days.

Nearly a week after our arrival I made my first domiciliary visit outside the village on Lancaster, to see a lady believed to be in labour ten miles away. When I got there I found she had been delivered a month before but did have a pelvic abscess requiring treatment.

After our first month at Ha Chooko we had more patients, many of them suffering from more serious problems as confidence grew. It was frustrating treating some of these necessarily as out patients when about 5% of all consultations would have benefited greatly from hospital care.

One day I was on my own in the dispensary when a whole gang of red ochre-smeared young men suddenly converged on the dispensary making a tremendous noise – I really thought my time had come and quickly locked the door and hid beneath the examination couch. It transpired that this was a visit from an initiation school and one of their number had got badly infected following circumcision and they had wisely brought him for treatment. I gave him a long acting injection of penicillin and advised him to bathe every day in the river.

Arnold and I began to attend a weekly clinic each Friday in a small room at the trading store across the river which had previously been used by Dr. Carl Van Aswegan who came up from the lowlands. Our first visit there was on a very wet day and we slithered and slipped our way there down to the river and up to the store. We only had five patients owing to the torrential rain. This was a relief as we were still awaiting some essential medical supplies to be brought up on the lorry from Maseru.

After 10 days at Ha chooko I first felt 'home sick' 4 ½ months after leaving England. This soon passed after I had been to mass and remembered all those whom we knew were praying for us.

In addition to our dispensary in the village and the clinic at the store, on the 19th July I took over as Government Medical Officer at the Health Centre, Ha Marakabei – 12 miles down the mountain road. This involved holding a busy weekly clinic with a resident Mosotho nurse and doing necessary post-mortem examinations. The later were time consuming as they usually necessitated a trip to Maseru to give court evidence. When our one vehicle was occupied I rode on Lancaster to Marakabei. On one occasion I was late returning and as I descended from the hospital site to get to Ha Chooko the light suddenly went and there was no moon. Thinking my horse would find his way home I gave him his head. However, Lancaster had other ideas and went and found some luscious grass in the valley and then I found myself back at the hospital site. Fortunately one of our workers who was sleeping in the corrugated iron store we were erecting on the south side of the hospital site, heard me and was happy to guide me back to Ha Chooko by the aid of the mission mule. After that I always carried a powerful torch in the saddle-bag.

I was asked to go and take charge of the Government Hospital at Mokhotlong at the foot of the Drakensberg for a week, as the lone doctor there was suddenly taken ill. This involved going down to Maseru and then flying to Mokhotlong in a two-seater Cessna plane. This was a foretaste of things to come and I enjoyed seeing another mountain hospital at close quarters. My return flight proved to be the fright of my life when we just could not get over the Maloti Mountains due to strong wind and rain. The pilot said we would have to return to Mokhotlong as we were running short of fuel! We successfully completed a further attempt when the weather settled down that same afternoon at 4pm.

While I had been away Arnold had coped extremely well on his own but was glad to see me back.

August proved to be a very windy month but Gerry managed to get the roof on the hospital store, which was quite an accomplishment. We continued at Ha Chooko and coped with numerous lacerations and fractures. One day a man called Thibelo Mpee arrived with a severely infected eye and there was a grave risk that this might affect his other eye. This involved removing the infected eye under sedation and local anaesthetic using some improvised instruments. My venture into major opthalmic surgery went well and I was later able to get him a glass eye, which proved a great novelty in the Maloti.

By Mid August we had formulated a draft plan for the future hospital which the hospital board eventually accepted with a few modifications. In early September we cared for a temporary in-patient at the dispensary. She had dislocated her knee and could not possibly be dealt with as an out-patient. At our first domiciliary midwifery case in the village, we delivered a baby boy whom they called Kenneth – poor chap!

Our store at the hospital site was completed and we decided that a pre-fabricated three- bedroom dwelling would be the next job so that we could go and live on-site as soon as possible. When the parts of the prefab were unloaded from the lorry they were numbered A-Z for easy assembly but so many parts were so badly damaged in transit from Maseru and nearly every pane of glass was broken and had to be replaced. Arnold and Gerry worked like Trojans straightening and assembling the metal parts amazingly well and completed our future dwelling.

Cement blocks were made on site using local labour as the expense of transporting ready made ones would have been prohibitive. Cement was brought up by lorry from Maseru and sand had to be fetched from the Senqunyane river 10 miles down the Mountain Road, as the sand in the Mantšonyane river was unsuitable. The water required was initially obtained from a spring a ¼ mile away near the Trader's house and fetched in 44 gallon drums by Land Rover. Enough cement blocks were made in this way to build a two-roomed clinic close to the prefab for use as soon as we moved across to take up residence at the hospital site. Several traditional rondavels were erected to house the ground staff, and by the end of February 1962 we were ready to leave Ha Chooko and centralise our activities on the hospital site which had been fenced and measured almost a mile in perimeter.

During our time at Ha Chooko we had treated well over 1000 patients, performed 100 or so minor operations and attended 100 antenatal cases and a few actual deliveries. Patients arrived at all hours of the day or night having travelled for one to two days to reach us. In addition I was called out about three times a week to visit the sick at home – sometimes several hours ride on horseback. Sometimes a horse would be brought for me to ride , but after developing severe sciatica from a worn out saddle I always insisted on using my own saddle. We managed to procure some of the old style saddles used by the Basutoland Mounted Police. These were extremely comfortable with a deep seat and well suited to long mountain treks when one could sit back and let the horse clamber over rocks. We never had our horses shod as wet rocks could be a great hazard. Over the years I treated a number of Mounted Police with head injuries, as they had to shoe their horses because they were used so much.

Occasionally I had to spend the night on the mud floor of a rondavel, if a call came late in the day when there was no moon. I always preferred well used mud floors to lie on because it was less smoky with an indoor fire and over time there were smoothed contours which seemed to accommodate comfortably to the human anatomy. The offer of an ancient, possibly flea infested, mattress and bed was graciously declined. We were sorry to leave the village community and mission but it was time to move on.

Chapter 3 THE FIRST PHASE OF BUILDING

' A wise person …. built on solid rock' (Mt.7.24 CEV)

On the 5th March 1962 we moved our domicile after 9 months at Ha Chooko, to our new prefabricated dwelling on the hospital site. This involved taking our goods, chattels and medical supplies down the mountain, across the river and up to the more exposed plateau where the store/stable/workshop had been completed on the nearer south side of the site above the river and further on to the north side, our future home which awaited us on the north side of the small road we had made to link up with the quarter of a mile track to the Trading Store.

During the previous week men and women from Ha Chooko had each day taken over quite a lot of stuff on their way to work. I was up at 5:30am doing last minute packing and eventually went over at 2:30pm on Lancaster with a cardboard box containing our two Siamese cats we had inherited from Father Clement, when he had returned to the U.K after 5 years of hard work. Our Golden Labrador puppy had already gone over with Arnold and Gerry. Our removal was successfully completed apart from a trunk of Arnold's records arriving filled with river water. We soon felt at home in our new house, which Father Donald came over and blessed next day on Shrove Tuesday.

Thus began what we called Phase One of the hospital. We first had to prepare the temporary dispensary and were able to hold our first clinic on the fourth day after moving. We used the right hand room for consultations and the left-hand room as a dispensary and treatment room. It was only about 20 yards from our residence and so we could see patients arriving at odd times, as they often did.

Three weeks after we had moved I was delighted to serve our first Sesotho Mass celebrated by Father Donald in our store/workshop. We used the carpenters bench as an altar and celebrated the Annunciation. Twenty people attended this first service with great reverence in such humble surroundings – but after all, our Lord was a carpenter!

As one of our first major tasks we launched a massive immunisation programme against Diphtheria and Whooping Cough. Whooping Cough had caused many fatalities in our first winter and we were determined to complete at least 1000 immunisations before the coming winter. To accomplish this we visited schools far and near to which mothers brought their babies to be immunised together with all the school children. A quarter of these were carried out on two visits to Ha Nyane at the Roman Mission School of Auray, four miles further along the track. The effect of this campaign was a marked success as a preventative measure and we got to know most of the schools in the area on our visits to each of them. What is more, they got to know us.

Early in April we planted fir trees around the periphery of the site to act as a windbreak and we had our second in-patient with a fractured upper arm and skull. We accommodated him of necessity in the consultation room of the dispensary for a couple of days. That month proved our busiest yet with 250 new patient attendances and 150 old ones plus about 350 at the Marakabei Health Centre. We no longer needed to have a clinic at the Store and visited Ha Chooko once a week.

Soon after taking up residence on the site the foundations of the first phase of the hospital were laid. The foundations did not involve very much work because we were building on solid rock with little soil or grass to clear away. This first block was to be 110 feet long by 25 feet wide, running North to South with the front entrance facing West. A bulge on the centre of the East side was 30 feet by 20 feet and was to be the kitchen from the start. A corridor was to run the length of the building and connect all the rooms, which were designed with an intended future use but also for alternative temporary use pending the planned second phase of the building. The entrance hall and future waiting room was to accommodate four male beds. The southern half of the block was to include; in the future consulting room accommodation for three children's cots and four baby basinettes, in the future doctor's office a twin bedded delivery room and in the future operating theatre accommodation for five female beds. We would thus be able to take up to 16 in-patients. The northern half of the block was to include a treatment room to be used initially as a consulting room, a dispensary to serve at first for treatment, a store-room and a linen room as well.

Before any of this miniature hospital could be built we had to make 8000 cement blocks on-site. To accomplish this before the winter snows were upon us in June was our main objective. We employed a dozen or more unskilled men from the villages to help make the cement blocks which were made of 1 in 8 mixture of cement and sand. We were still fetching 250 gallons of water a day ¼ mile from the spring whilst waiting for the well to be finished and connected to the pipeline we had laid. We encountered great problems in digging the well. The pump gave a lot of trouble and an underground stream washed silt into the well almost as fast as the digging removed it. We also employed a number of women who happily smashed rocks from morn till night for future concrete making. Eventually, Mr. Clifford, a beneficent South African builder in Maseru, lent us a stone- crusher free of charge which proved much quicker.

All this work was organised and supervised by Gerry who had the difficult job of liasing with the building sub-committee in Maseru mainly via the store radio, often with bad atmospherics. We were fortunate in acquiring the services of a trained Mosotho builder called Egbert Jason Monese on whom we increasingly relied over the years. He was a short man of slight build with a small greying head and ready smile. He spoke excellent English and was a loyal and energetic worker. Although a committed member of the Lesotho Evangelical Church he was proud to tell you that he helped to build the new Roman Catholic Cathedral in Maseru as well as parts of their Mission at Ha

Marakabei, Egbert's home. At 54 years of age Egbert was extremely agile and insisted on doing everything at the double. He worked long hours and was always on call for emergencies. Only once a year could he be persuaded to have a day off to visit his home on one of our horses. Egbert's rich deep bass voice always led the singing as he, like many Basotho, read tonic soh-fa.

Egbert's right hand man was a skinny man of about the same age called Jacote Thene with whom Egbert worked very well. The leader of the cement block brigade was John Maseli. Under his stimulus at least 100 cement blocks a day were made. John had worked in the diamond mines at Kimberly in South Africa and no manual task, however difficult, ever proved beyond his strength and capability. He was illiterate but highly intelligent and had a marvellous sense of humour. He was also church warden at Ha Chooko and at a church meeting spoke so fast I usually caught only the occasional bits of wisdom with which he enthused the congregation. With the added help of a party of St Andrews' schoolboys from Bloemfontein with their master, Father Derek Damant (later Bishop of George in South Africa), enough cement blocks were made to enable building to begin. The actual walls were completed in about five weeks with the help of the two Portuguese builders working with our local team, and by the first of June, the first anniversary of our arrival, the roof trusses were in place. It was an impressive sight on turning the bend in the track from the store or riding over the nek to see a large grey structure looming up suddenly from the plateau with the village of Ha Chooko in the background. Each cement block had cost us about 15 shillings to make which meant that £6000 was spent before any building was done and more like £10000 was to be spent before completion and furnishing. Two thirds of Miss Pursers bequest had then been used but there was something to see and use by the end of September 1962.

Out-patient attendances continued to increase and Arnold seemed to cope well on his own if I had to be away and became quite efficient with dental extractions and minor surgery, which not many nurses then did.

Sadly, Gerry had to leave us after 18 months of very hard and demanding work, both physically and emotionally, and return to the UK. He put so much into his work, which took a lot out of him. All who realised the hazards and problems of the initial building felt a great debt of gratitude for all that Gerry had accomplished as a key man in such a short time against almost impossible odds. For the time being Arnold had to relinquish medical and nursing duties and turn his hand to building liaison and administration.

For the time being I was then left to work pretty much on my own apart from the help of Martin Moejane whom I began to train to make up mixtures in the dispensary, accurately dispense medications and give clear instructions to patients. I could now manage fairly well without his help in translation but would occasionally have to seek his help with a knotty problem through the hatch between the examination room and the dispensary.

The variety of medical cases extended by the week. I performed my first forceps delivery on the mud floor of a rondavel just down the Mountain Road. This was at the home of 'Mamankoto, a traditional Mosotho doctor called a Bone-Thrower (Selaoli), who uses a set of stones, shells and engraved bones which are cast on the floor to diagnose and treat illnesses and troubles according to the position in which they fall. No sooner was the baby delivered when 'Mamankoto began throwing the bones beside me and I had no idea of the significance at the time. She obviously approved of me to allow me to be called to deliver her grandchild whom she named after me and so I could hardly disapprove of her. In fact this was the beginning of a mutual respect I developed with traditional doctors of several kinds. 'Mamankoto herself actually came to the hospital some years later suffering from advanced liver disease for which, unfortunately, I was able to do little.

Towards the end of July Egbert carefully wired the roof trusses against the August gales. In a few days the Portuguese builders completed the corrugated iron roof. The 13th August was a red-letter day when water first gushed forth from the plastic piping onto the hospital site from the well ¼ of a mile away. The long delay in completing the well with great difficulties meant that our Land Rover was in a very sad state after transporting all the water for building phase one. We therefore traded it in for a ¾ ton GMC pickup with three gears. This was a comfortable vehicle to drive but was quite hair raising to drive in the wet season and almost impossible in the heavy snow. The plastering of the internal walls was accomplished by two South African builders from Maseru in less than 2 months and by the end of September the hospital floor had been laid.

On the 27th September 1962 although far from ready, we had to nurse our very first in-patient, Alphonsi Sekola, with advanced Tuberculosis Peritonitis for the last three weeks of his life. Our second patient to stay also suffered from Tuberculosis. He was Josepha Matsie, a young emaciated boy, whom we were able to discharge after 3 months in a picture of health and vitality, able to continue his treatment as an outpatient. It really was quite amazing how quickly and well tuberculosis patients responded to treatment – we encountered no problems with drug resistance and were able to cure many cases in a matter of months rather than years.

Building a hospital on rock foundation, in biblical fashion, was fine; but we are not told how the wise person coped with sanitary requirements and water supply. By the end of November Mr. Cloete, an elderly but charming South African, completed the Septic Tank and French drain for our prefab; but the French drains for the hospital proved extremely difficult for lack of depth of soil and very hard rock. We were fearful of dynamiting in case we weakened what was already built. However, with perseverance and heavy manual work the drainage was completed. The water supply problem had still not been solved. It soon became clear that the supply we had struggled to establish would not be sufficient for future requirements in the dry season –

expert advice from the geological point of view had been over-optimistic. We therefore had to look elsewhere for an additional supply down in the valley to the east of the hospital. On measuring this spring even during the driest month of September it was producing 2,700 gallons per day and furthermore we were assured by local residents that it had not dried up even in the severe drought of 1933 when villages all around had used it. The new spring was only about half the distance of the old one; the disadvantage being that we had to pump up about 150 feet and use more fuel.

By the end of December, 18 months after our arrival, we were able to have a hot bath! We had treated 5000 patients and had been amazed at the variety of complaints that confronted us. Arnold and I had extracted between us 200 teeth many of which involved much blood and sweat due to the advanced state of caries often present. Patients had been very conscientious at attending for courses of treatment and Whooping Cough had caused much less mortality thanks to our immunisation programme. I had had to perform my first tracheotomy for Diphtheria - Egbert helped as Arnold was away. I also treated a local school teacher for alcohol addiction by means of hypnosis and he did very well.

Our cultivated land backing on to the road had been ploughed and sown. We had new potatoes and peas for Christmas. We had planted more trees; poplars, some fruit trees and 300 acorns. The latter were something of an experiment at 7000 feet (there are no Oak trees today!). We planted Red Hot Pokers along the entrance drive in the hope they might thrive. Several rondavels were built to accommodate waiting ante-natal ladies and also Tuberculosis patients who lived too far away to attend for regular injections. We began using a rondavel as a temporary chapel for morning Sesotho prayers. Egbert began to read for us and soon grew in confidence.

Early in the new year of 1963 Chief Chooko, having recently ridden over to see how we were getting on, died at the age of 83. I'm sure he had wanted to be our first proper in-patient; but this was not to be. Even so he did see the beginning of the realisation of Bishop John's promise made to him 12 years earlier, taking visible shape and this bought tears to his eyes. A requiem was sung in our little chapel for him.

Mr. Cloete pressed ahead with shelving in the hospital; carried out cement work and painting of the outside walls, including the huge white cross surrounded by red Italian plaster as a contrasting background. By this time water was connected to the hospital and we were using flush toilets. I became quite expert on minor running repairs to the flushing mechanisms as they always seemed to go wrong when no-one else was available.

I extracted a very septic tooth under hypnosis in Sesotho and led Sesotho prayers for the first time in our rondavel chapel. However, there were less pleasant jobs such as doing post-mortems for the Government. These were mainly assault cases, especially fractured skulls due to heavy blows from a *knobkerrie*, but some were accidental deaths.

On one occasion I was called over to Ha Chooko by the Mounted Police to examine a man who had hanged himself with a grass rope from a large rock. The Police were sent for without disturbing the scene of the apparent suicide. Meanwhile the man untied the rope and walked into the hut in the dead of night. When I arrived, just after the policeman, the man was very much alive and sitting with handcuffs on!

At the end of January we welcomed Peter Parker as general handyman and building supervisor. He was 26 years old and had served some years in the Royal Engineers and had worked in East Africa for 3 years. Peter was much at home with horses and was a qualified radio mechanic. It then became possible for Arnold to resume nursing duties, which was a great help to me. Our new man, Peter, lost no time in completing the power-house in which we installed a 6KW Lister engine and the electrical fittings.

On 28th March we first had electric light in the prefab from dusk until 10pm. A large paraffin deep freezer came up by lorry but we had enormous difficulty getting it into the hospital kitchen. Another marathon task involved hoisting up 3 large water storage tanks onto 24 foot platforms for the hospital water supply.

On 15th April our first African staff nurse arrived. She was Pauline Ebuse Sixishe. With her 15 stones she cut a striking picture of a woman of great dignity with a pale yellow-brown complexion, twinkling eyes and broad Negroid nose. She was a true Masotho inspite of her Xhosa surname through marriage. She had been educated at St Catherine's in Maseru, the Anglican Teachers Training College. She had gone on to train as a nurse at the Bargwaneth hospital in Johannesburg. Pauline was keen to serve her own people, which she was to do with dedication, hard work and good humour for the rest of her life.

On the day following Pauline's arrival we moved from the temporary dispensary by the prefab into the hospital building. On that day a younger staff nurse called Elginia Ncqugana arrived late at night on the bus in a half frozen state. Pauline and Elginia shared a rondavel at first. Together they did a marvellous job in those first few months when one or the other was always on call.

Pauline quickly became a mother figure in whom the patients placed an implicit trust. They would knock her up at any hour of the day or night and she would come and tap ever so lightly on my bedroom window, gradually increasing the intensity until I was roused (far pleasanter than being rudely awakened by the telephone). We spent many night hours together stitching up wounds, plastering fractures and delivering difficult babies. Pauline was a great support and never seemed to tire of helping those in need. She could at times be quite firm when required but mostly she was the essence of patience and gentleness. During the five years I had the pleasure of working with Pauline I relied on her tact and ability to translate in any situation which required sensitivity. She was the only interpreter I ever felt confident in using in such situations. She knew precisely what you meant and put it into the most beautiful and idiomatic Sesotho. Pauline was never happier than in the outpatient department with the mothers-to-be or the babies and children.

Elginia being younger and slimmer soon showed what she lacked in experience she compensated for in enthusiasm. She didn't mind being packed off on a horse for domiciliary visits or home deliveries if I was otherwise engaged. Elginia had only one fall from a rather obstreperous horse.

On June 1st 1963 we celebrated the second anniversary of our arrival in the Maloti by admitting our first patient into the hospital under full nursing supervision and care. She was suffering from pneumonia. The next day our first male patient was admitted after being kicked by a horse. In the early hours of 3rd June Elginia delivered our first hospital baby, an 8lb-baby boy called 'Tsietse' (Trouble)!

Arnold became nursing supervisor and in charge of stores. We appointed an initial domestic staff consisting of cook, washerwoman and two domestics. Our cook Juliata was an obese lady with a pleasant smile. She was so obese that it was impossible to observe when she became pregnant. We were never made privy to such information for her fear that she might lose her job. We usually managed to whisk her of to the delivery room minutes before the arrival of her babies and she was back at work within a few weeks.

Juliata had quite a difficult task in making the food go round. We were never quite certain how much of this was due to the importunity of frequent hungry visitors or Juliata's own insatiable appetite. We soon learned the wisdom of a lockable receptacle for essential foods and that it was best to weigh out each commodity required for the day. A strict ban on all visitors to the kitchen also became a prudent necessity. Thus a marked economy on food supply was effected but no one went hungry.

The other extravagance was the 'Aga' type solid fuel oven, which was always stoked up to tropical heat levels and proved a source of great attraction to all hospital workers. I don't think we ever achieved a realistic economy on fuel. At least the premature babies seemed to thrive well in the hot humid atmosphere above the kitchen oven!.

Rebecca and Flora were responsible for cleaning, washing and ironing. Rebecca Lekolomi proved a most conscientious and industrious worker; but her colleague, Flora, seemed to disappear for long intervals and was often found curled up in some odd place – sometimes in the patients' bath!

The hospital at this stage looked quite attractive as one approached. The cream walls and blue window frames and fascia board formed a pleasant contrast with the greens and browns of the surrounding countryside. The doors were varnished and the front door surmounted by the huge white cross on its dark red background.

Bishop John was keen that we should have a small hospital chapel. SPG agreed to fund this and Dennis Hall was sent up to build the chapel which took him about six weeks to complete. Egbert built a free-standing altar from beautiful purple stones gathered from nearly a mile down the mountain road.

On Saturday 7th September we had the official opening of St. James' hospital by his Honour the Resident Commissioner, Mr. (later Sir) Alexander Giles. CMG, MBE. The King of Lesotho, Moshoeshoe II., was hoping to attend but was indisposed at the last minute; but sent a message with his representative Chief Reentseng Griffiths. Convoys of cars streamed up the Mountain Road and about 1000 Basotho from the surrounding district converged on the hospital.

After welcoming our guests I said: 'Today is a landmark in the progress of Basutoland and in the life of the Maloti.' At 7am that morning our chapel had been dedicated at a sung mass with 70 people present, by Bishop John in honour of 'The Divine Compassion and St. Barnabas'. The reason for the title was suggested by learning that the old name for the hospital site was 'Khaula' (A place of compassion or a nice place). Our fervent hope was that the hospital would, as the years went by, continue to reflect something of the divine compassion of our Lord for his suffering people; like Barnabas 'the Son of Consolation'.

Bishop John pointed out that: 'this hospital has been built by the Anglican Church and is served by it; but it is for all who need its services. Most of the money has come from members of the Church in England through the SPG, but there had been generous donations from the Anglo American Corporation, De Beers and the Native Recruitment Corporation.'

Bishop John particularly thanked the devoted and hard working members of the Executive Committee of the hospital's governing body especially Mr. Neil Yeats as chairman, Mr. Mervyn Barnes and Mr. Charles Barry, who had been fairly frequent visitors during the building process (they were keen fishermen!). He also thanked Mr. Colin Unsworth who had drawn up all the plans free of charge.

Mr. Neil Yates paid tribute to all who had worked to achieve so much under the difficult conditions of the past two years. He also urged the people of Mantšonyane to take the hospital to their hearts and give it all their possible support in the coming years.

The King's message said:

'Convey our greetings to all the people of Mantšonyane. Tell them how grateful we are for the boon of the hospital. A great debt is owed to the members of the Anglican Church and to all the supporters in Britain who have contributed to the construction of the hospital. This reminds me of the Great Moshoeshoe who placed us under the protection of her Majesty's Government'.

The Resident Commissioner said that for three centuries Christianity and medicine had been closely associated in many places. He recalled driving over the mountains at Braemar in his native Scotland, when he negotiated a steep pass, known as 'Devil's Elbow', and came to the head of the Glen where there is a place called 'The Spital of Glenshiel' – there was a hospital there run by the church in the Middle Ages. Here, then was the Spital of Mantšonyane, which he hoped would be treasured by the people. Mr. Giles adapted the Royal Air Force motto (*Per ardua ad alta*) to 'Per ardua ad Aspirin' which the interpreter rendered as 'Through the steep places to find medicine!' His honour was presented with a silver key and unveiled a commemorative plaque in the entrance hall.

Bishop John then blessed the hospital from outside the front entrance wearing cope and mitre and chanting the blessing in Sesotho. We sang 'Pleasant are they Courts above' and then the Sesotho National Anthem (*Lesotho, fatše la bontata' rona*) – 'Lesotho, land of our fathers'.

The flying Doctor Carl Vanaswegn dropped congratulatory leaflets as he flew over us.

There followed a buffet lunch for visitors from Maseru and a massive feast (*mokete*) for the people with a large Ox roast and gallons of Sesotho beer (*Joala*), made by the Mother's Union of Ha Chooko. It was a memorable day enjoyed by all. We quietly said Compline in our new chapel before collapsing into bed.

Next day we had Sesotho prayers in the chapel for the first time. A week later we fixed up a suspended ploughshare to use as a bell and rang the Angelus for the first time. I plucked up courage and preached a short Sesotho sermon on the following Sunday. On the following day it was back to harsh reality. After being up all night with diarrhoea I had to ride 11 hours to attend a lady with a retained placenta. On the 22nd September we held our first service for patients in the hospital itself and I delivered my first baby whom we called Martha, the name of a great aunt and one of my mother's names.

The Basotho liked to have an English name as well as a Sesotho name. One could often guess the denomination of a baby. The French Protestants often had Old Testament names like Azariah while the Roman Catholic ones were often saddled with the name of a Pope such as Pius. Anglicans tended to go for New Testament names such as Elisabetha or Maria.

We cared for a herd boy with the Sesotho name *Lefa* ('Inheritance') Matseke who was paralysed down his right side due to an injury. During the month he was with us Arnold gave him daily physiotherapy and to our delight he left hospital on his own two feet, fully recovered.

Another boy was Maqoma Ramoe (the 'q' is a click sound and is pronounced by making contact with the tongue on the roof of the mouth and quickly withdrawing it). The clicks were probably copied from the Bushmen, the original inhabitants of Lesotho, who were absorbed by the Basotho. Maqoma was brought a 6-hour ride from Ha Mohapeloa with a fractured femur. We decided that he was small enough to be treated by the 'Gallows Method' which meant suspending him by his feet with his buttocks raised just above the bed. This method, normally only used for children under three worked well for Maqoma although he was 5 years old.

In October our life was somewhat disrupted when Brian Salt and Ian Struthers arrived to shoot a film about the hospital for SPG. It took a full week and Egbert Monese agreed to be the star patient whom I visited at home and who was strapped to a horse to come to the hospital for surgery. There were hair-raising shots as we galloped along a mountain path. It looked far more dangerous than it was as Ian took the shots from below and we were confident of the sure-footedness of our horses. It was all good fun and helped to give our supporters some idea of the setting in which we worked.

Shortly after this Alphonsina was brought to the hospital in a slightly agitated and paranoid state. We were told she had been 'bewitched' by a traditional doctor but it was very difficult to obtain an accurate history. We gently sedated her and laid hands on her with prayers, as the Fathers were away on trek. Next day she had completely recovered, made her confession and received Holy Communion.

Peter began to extend the original clinic, close to the prefab, to make it into a cottage for the expected arrival of our Matron in 3 months time.

By 1st November 1963, we had been open for five months, during which time we had admitted 80 patients, the number having increased month by month. Soon we admitted our first diabetic, Justina, who had to commence insulin injections. I had to lecture the nurses about this fairly rare condition in the Maloti.

Our first patient with Typhoid Fever was a little girl who quickly responded to treatment. Later we had to cope with an epidemic of Typhoid due to contaminated, unprotected village springs. Some Typhoid patients had unwisely been treated with enemas by traditional doctors. We tried to immunise the whole village where these people came from.

We were encouraged to install a Stevenson's Screen to establish a mini-meteorological station and Arnold took over regular readings for the Government. The hottest time in the mountains was usually around Christmas-time and so we tended to have our main celebration in the cool of the evening.

On 20th January 1964 Miss Dorothy Clare Withers arrived to be our first Matron (*Nese e Kholo* or 'Big Nurse'). Dorothy was a veteran missionary nurse of considerable experience. She had trained at Bristol as a nurse and midwife and then had taken the Orthopaedic Nursing Certificate at the Woodland's Hospital in Birmingham. Dorothy then went on to the College of the Ascension at Selly Oak for missionary training. In her early days she served in Portuguese East Africa where she gained great proficiency in the art of improvisation and administering a medical service well off the beaten track. At times she had worked without the services of a Doctor for long periods and even had to amputate legs savaged by crocodile bites. Fortunately there were no crocodiles in Lesotho, although there obviously had been where the Basotho originated as the major clan to which the King belonged was the *Bakoena* (crocodiles).

Dorothy Withers came to work with us at just the right time. She could make something out of almost nothing. Her experience was quite invaluable and for her age she was remarkably energetic – although suffering from osteo-arthritis of the hips. Most nurses of her vintage would have gracefully retired rather than come up to St. James' and start all over again. Dorothy laid firm foundations in the development of nursing and administration. She proved the most marvellous deputy for me and I had no need to worry when away from the hospital – I knew Dorothy could cope with any problem without flinching. Her diagnostic and therapeutic skills were excellent; she could do quite a lot of surgery and could manage quite difficult deliveries. I was often glad of her orthopaedic expertise.

Although our new matron had not ridden a horse for many years, she never failed to ride over to Ha Chooko to church every Sunday unless the river was in flood or heavy snow made it impossible to go.

Dorothy soon made herself at home in her cottage complete with kitchen and bathroom. She called it 'Eaglet's Nest'. She could often be seen hobbling around with her rubber tipped walking stick, to and fro around the hospital. She got on well with the staff nurses and began training some local girls as Nurse Aids to assist in the hospital. These girls proved very keen and took Red Cross certificates in nursing and first aid.

A very popular baby clinic was started on Wednesdays when I was usually down at the Marakabei Health Centre – so I missed the squawking babies and their doting mothers who were soon competing with each other for the best fed and dressed infant. Dorothy would pick out ill babies to be seen on my return. In similar vein she was always the first to spot a waiting patient with Typhoid Fever – she was never wrong in her spot diagnosis.

Shortly after Dorothy's arrival Arnold was able to go on home-furlough. A week later Peter completed a year's service of great value on the building side and saw phase one brought to completion.

By 1st June 1964, our third anniversary of arrival, we had been operating as a functioning hospital for a year and had admitted 268 patients for periods of a week or longer. Chest and Midwifery cases were easily the commonest causes for admission. We had on average of at least nine patients staying but sometimes double this number with a few improvised beds. Most patients were women and children but we had a few men who needed to stay for long periods. It had been wonderful to see the results of good feeding especially with children.

One of our long stay patients was a young shepherd whose face had been struck by lightning and badly lacerated – he was lucky not to have been killed. S/N Pauline admitted him and shook her head without saying that she thought he was not long for this world. But he was a strong man and when he had recovered from the initial shock we carried out numerous operations on his face which really had to be re-fashioned. Due as much to his remarkable ability to heal as my skills as a plastic surgeon; he was able to leave hospital in a few weeks with a new face.

Our fourth winter proved to be a hard one when we were cut off from Maseru by snow for three weeks at a time and all the water pipes froze solid with no hot baths. It was a difficult time but the hardy Basotho kept us cheerful.

Being more established, calls to the outlying villages became less frequent but I often rode to Marakabei on my new horse called *Tšeliso* even when the road was not passable with a vehicle. Tšeliso had I believe been a race-horse in the Orange Free State at one time. He could still move fast and with a comfortable gait. He could cover 25 miles in less than three hours which is fast for the Maloti.

On June 14th we kept the patronal festival of our chapel 3 days late, with a Sung Mass and Procession with 100 people present. After a slide show we finished with Solemn Evensong and Te Deum. Regular Morning and Evening Prayers were started soon after with staff taking a full part in leading, reading and singing.

On 4th July we suspended a large wooden cross above the altar and on the following day Father Donald brought the Blessed Sacrament over from Ha Chooko to be kept in an aumbry immediately behind the free-standing altar. At 4:30pm we sang Benediction (*Tumeliso*). It was wonderful to have the Sacramental Presence of Our Lord with us and readily available for sick communions.

Father Harker arrived from St. Andrew's School, Bloemfontein with a further party of schoolboys to build us a foot suspension bridge across the Mantšonyane River. This was to be 200 feet down stream from where we usually crossed and needed to span 100 feet. Forty Rands, a gift from Edith Wilson, covered the cost of ropes and timber and the job was completed in 4 days. Matron Dorothy and S/N Pauline were the first to cross the bridge.

On 14th July the plot for the doctor's house was marked out and on 30th July Dr James Rawes arrived from St. Peter's Madinare in Bechuanaland to cover my home furlough for 6 months. Arnold returned from his furlough on 2nd August and I left 2 days later to fly home on 11th August 1964.

We had completed phase one of the hospital but phase two was to be built. I visited many parishes in the South of England and some elsewhere to encourage further support that was going to be required to finish the wards and operating theatre. There were already sufficient funds for the phase two building but I was glad to learn that further assistance would be forthcoming for essential equipment through a continuation of the projects scheme of SPG from the supporting parishes in England.

CHAPTER 4. THE SECOND PHASE OF BUILDING.

'We must be careful how we build' (1 Cor. 3.10b. CEV)

Towards the end of my furlough in England, just before Christmas 1964, I married Hazel, a geography teacher whom I had known for many years. Six weeks after our wedding I was due to return to Mantšonyane and we made a very difficult decision: that Hazel would complete teaching her 'A-Level' students until the end of the summer term. She would then rejoin me at the end of July, when we would have a house of our own at the hospital ready for habitation. During my stay in England I had secured the promise of a Land Rover Ambulance from the people of Dunchurch Rural Deanery in Coventry Diocese. This was to be fully fitted out and sent to us as a really necessary and useful help. It would make patient transport so much easier. Many sick people would face a much shorter journey on horseback and some who needed to go to the Queen Elizabeth II hospital in Maseru would have a far more comfortable journey down the Mountain Road.

On my return on the 14th February 1965 I was welcomed with a tea party. I was delighted that the second phase of building, started in September 1964 after I had left, was now well advanced. We had decided to contract out this work to Mr. Clifford, a South African, who had done much building in Maseru. The second phase of building consisted of an extension at both ends of the hospital. On the south end was a Delivery Theatre and a small Isolation Ward. On the north end a Matron's office, an X-ray and Darkroom together with a small Laboratory. At right angles to the southern end was a south wing comprising a twenty bedded Female Ward to be equipped by and named after the six donor parishes of Bromsgrove, Worcestershire, with two smaller contiguous Wards for Children and Men. The Children's Ward was to be called Bexhill Ward as this parish in Kent was to furnish it. The Male Ward was named after Buckingham, our much loved horse, who died from 'staggers' by eating Ragwort whilst on loan to a nameless person who didn't realise that a horse on trek had to be fed regularly! Buckinghamshire was of course the home of our builder of phase one, Gerald Garroway.

Bexhill and Buckingham Wards provided a further fifteen beds between them. We hit on the idea that a sliding door between the wards would allow flexibility of occupancy between children and men – there would probably be more children than men most of the time. We were looking forward to having thirty-five beds in all.

The temporary wards were overflowing when I returned to the hospital and took over again from Dr. James Rawes who had held things together very well for 6 months. He left us to go and work in Zambia. The doctor's house was also well advanced at this time. I had two sleepless nights when my mind wouldn't switch off, thinking about the hundreds of questions to be answered in getting the hospital organised. But after that I was so busy that there was no time for insomnia. Matron Dorothy and Arnold were of great support and we set to work, not only with all the practicalities of equipping phase two, but also trying to plan our patient care wisely and sensibly according to the resources of staff available.

By June the new wards were completed and came into full use. It was good to be able to nurse patients more easily and marvellous to have a sluice room and a bathroom for patients. We thus commemorated the fourth anniversary of arrival at Mantšonyane and second anniversary of admitting in-patients by moving into the more spacious wards. This allowed us to use the entrance hall as a waiting room and have an outpatient consulting room instead of using the treatment room. Both doctor and matron now had the luxury of an office of their own. The operating theatre could now be equipped and put into use in memory of Mary Maund, wife of Bishop John.

It took five months to replace our second staff nurse, as having been to town for training, nurses were reluctant to return to the isolation of the mountains. There were unforeseen problems concerning the standard six girls we were training as Nurse Aids. We were told that women would not attend for hospital confinement as it was against Sesotho custom for an unmarried girl to assist while a woman was in labour. One man complained that we ought not use a nurse aid as an interpreter for matron in the ante-natal clinic. We took a firm but gentle stand about this problem and explained there was no alternative to using these young unmarried women, who within a short time would be mothers themselves. There never seemed to be any decrease in the number of Midwifery cases, which outnumbered all other patients and antenatal clinics increased week by week.

At the end of my first week back in harness, we held our first meeting of the Hospital Board on site at the hospital. It was good not to have to go down to Maseru and all members were keen to see the progress to date. On the same day Brother Hugh, who had joined Father Hector, who had replaced Father Don at Ha Chooko, completed the mammoth task of making a track that only a four wheel drive could use to get to St. James' Church and Mission at Ha Chooko. Even then there would be times with the river in full flood when they might still be cut off from us at the hospital. However, that year we experienced the worst drought in the Maloti for over thirty years. The staple crop of maize was dried up in the fields and the coming winter was likely to (and in fact did) produce a glut of malnutrition especially in the children and the elderly, together with an increased susceptibility to infection. This scenario made it imperative to increase our bed space and facilities as soon as possible.

On Easter Monday, I was called to Ha Toka to deliver a fine baby girl, who was to be called Paseka (Easter). To try and reduce time-consuming home deliveries we encouraged pregnant mothers from distant villages to come and live in the rondavels we had built at the hospital, at any time after seven months. They fed and looked after themselves (sometimes mother-in-law came too). This seemed to work quite well as a day or two's ride on horse-back in a highly pregnant state was always a problem and sometimes they gave birth on their way to us!

At the end of July I went down to Cape Town to meet my wife, Hazel and we enjoyed a second honeymoon at Sea Point before going back to Mantšonyane. On our arrival back at the hospital there was a great welcome for Hazel who was immediately named `Mathabo (Mother of Joy). My own Sesotho name was *Ramosa* (Father of Kindness) – a difficult one to live up to. The staff I found also called me *Thoso* (the one who appears from nowhere!). Egbert gave us a whole sheep as a belated wedding present. We soon got into some sort of routine in our new home. Hazel declined to have any domestic help but eventually let Rosa, Matron's domestic wash and iron the sheets which was all done by hand. We began the day with short prayers in chapel with the staff, followed by breakfast. Hazel usually joined us for coffee breaks in the hospital at mid-morning. I continued the Marakabei clinic on Wednesdays and tried to have a half-day on Thursdays. On alternate weekends Dorothy would cover for me so that there was a chance I might not be called, except for more major emergencies. Hazel began giving the Nurse Aids English lessons on Friday afternoons.

On 27th October the Land Rover Ambulance donated by Dunchurch arrived – a great jubilation accompanied this wonderful asset. There were a fair number of night calls – usually for midwifery.

By November the temperature dropped below freezing at night and the early peas and beans we had planted looked a sorry sight. This meant the most of the land had to be replanted to ensure a supply of greens for the patients. We also used to dry greens for the hospital for the winter months.

Hazel began keeping the accounts instead of me. Her arithmetic had always been better than mine and she always managed to balance the books.

It was good to celebrate Christmas by making a crib in the main ward so that patients, visitors and staff were able sing carols and have morning prayers. The Nurse Aids put on a Nativity play in the chapel and all but 3 in-patients managed to get along and really enjoyed the local talent. Normally staff shared morning and evening payers in chapel while the Senior Nurse on duty led ward prayers for the patients.

At the end of 1965 we felt that the hospital had become a reality after so much sweat and toil.

Early in January 1966 we were sorry to lose Arnold, who returned to England after 5 years devoted to the hospital in a variety of capacities – Nurse, Builder, Maintenance Man, Farmer, Store Keeper, Driver and general factotum of infinite resources. Above all he was a trusted colleague through thick and thin in the really hard work of getting St. James' Hospital established and overcoming tremendous initial difficulties.

Staff Nurse Pauline was still with us and was joined by a new staff nurse from the Scott Hospital, Morija in the lowland, called Alina Makamole. Our six Nurse Aids proved very keen to learn and gradually took on more responsibility. We engaged a Mosotho driver Johannes who also helped with building and odd jobs.

Our x-ray unit was a very good Australian portable machine and proved to be a tremendous help with chest x-rays of Tuberculosis patients and it also took very good skull and limb x-rays. The well-equipped dark room was a joy to work in.

We were pleased to participate in a preventative Health Week at Marakabei Clinic. I gave a talk on communicable diseases and Pauline gave forth on Maternal and Child Care. Other talks were on dental care, growing food and accidents in the home. In this first venture on health education in the area the Basotho who attended seemed very keen to learn and I'm sure it was all extremely worthwhile.

That summer was lovely with good rains to cool us down and a wonderful crop of wild mushrooms which were delicious to eat. The Mountain Road became difficult to negotiate without Four-Wheel drive. No lorry reached us for ten days with post and supplies. Fortunately, Matron Dorothy believed in stocking in enormous supplies so there were no real problems.

The storks in the valley were of great interest. They came from the rooftops of Germany and migrated each year to Lesotho via the Holy Land and always returned to Europe in March. That year, early one evening, John Maseli arrived on our stoep (verandah) proudly holding a stork by its legs. He had stealthily crept up on the poor bird, grabbed it and ended its life, never to return home. He excitedly told us that he had killed it 'because it was eating my crops!' He was surprised that I was not pleased with his proficiency. It was the only time I had reason to be cross with John; but he had acted in ignorance of the fact that storks only fed on insects that often harmed the crops. Our hospital Labrador, Judy, had a whale of a time, endlessly chasing the beautiful Long-tailed Widow Birds, which hovered over the crops in the valley. She was I am pleased to record, never successful in catching one.

At the end of March we decide to make a start on a cement block Nurses' Home to the rear of, but close to the hospital. Hitherto our Staff Nurses and Nurse Aids were living in rondavels and we thought it would be better to house them in more adequate quarters with flushing toilets and more spacious facilities. The Nurses Home design was simple but was capable of being made very comfortable. It was to be built in a 'U-Shape', about 50 yards behind the hospital. There was to be a central dining room and common room with a Kitchen on one side of it and a wash room on the other. Each of the two wings housed a large dormitory for three to four Nurse Aids with a smaller room on the ends for a staff nurse. A Covered stoep ran around the inner aspect. This would provide a sheltered area for sitting outside. We managed to obtain funds for this project amounting to £2,000 from the Mines Corporation. So far, so good: but who was to build it? I asked our trusted friend Egbert if he could build it on his own with local help. 'Yes of course' he replied without hesitation. This he did, in fact, extremely well. The only thing necessary was to check his measurements as the building proceeded. At coffee break I would sprint across from the hospital for this purpose each day and then sprint back to carry on with the out-patients' clinic.

The rains continued throughout the autumn. I had a very slippery ride to Ha Lebone to see a woman with pneumonia. On the return journey my guides horse's girth strap broke but I succeeded in repairing it with hair from the horses tail! 'There is usually an alternative use for everything' was a maxim that I proved time and time again in many difficult situations.

A teacher from Ha Leronti asked if he could pay his hospital fees in cabbages, which kept the hospital well-supplied for weeks; but matron complained about the smell from storing them.

In five weeks we were ready to put the roof trusses on the Nurses Home – not so bad for a DIY venture.

At that time we could buy a whole sheep for 6 Rands (£3) – when we first arrived, 5 years before, they were only 5 Rands (£2.50)! Mutton was our regular meat intake and we evolved different ways of using it, most popular of which was a curry with powder bought in bulk from an Indian market in Durban. One was called 'Hell Fire', another 'Masala Mix' and yet another 'Mother-in-law!' Beef was a rare delicacy and Pork was unknown in the mountains at that time. In the lowlands Rabbit was eaten especially in the French communities. Any change from mutton was always very welcome!

One Wednesday I decided not to visit Marakabei as usual as the sky looked like heavy rain and there would be very few patients. This was just as well as I had an urgent call to Ha Rankomo to a lady with a retained placenta (afterbirth). Had I gone as usual to Marakabei, it is more than likely she would have bled to death before I got to her. This was only one of many times when I felt guided to a course of action out of the routine, later discovering why.

In August we had to deal with a great number of old people with pneumonia. It was unusually a very windy month - which may have had something to do with this. I visited one man who claimed to be over 100 years old.

Early in September Henry Hardy arrived on the lorry from Maseru as a voluntary worker for 6 months. He was going up to Oxford the next year. We were very pleased with his ability with carpentry, which was well utilised in the hospital over the next few months. Other young men appeared from time to time and stayed sometimes for weeks. No charge was made for board or lodging. However, we usually managed to put their particular talents to good use. The right people so often appeared at the right time when a particular job needed to be done.

We acquired a dozen hens from the Agriculture Department – Rhode Island Reds and White Leghorns. They were laying well within three or four months, much to Hazel's delight.

Egbert's son got married and his father had to pay twenty cows, ten sheep and a horse to the bride's family – this was usual practice in the Maloti; as luck would have it Egbert had several sons all of whom had to provide a similar 'bride–price'. In real terms each son's wedding cost Egbert about R500 (£250). No wonder he worked so hard!

The first rains for four months began. Bishop John came and blessed the new wards on 26th September – they were full. There was a call in the early hours of the morning to a home delivery. I rode back at daybreak and then castrated the new Siamese Kittens in the hospital before snatching a few hours sleep! Other veterinary work was occasionally with horses. I learned the Sesotho method of giving a horse an enema by standing it with its forelegs on much higher ground with two strong Basotho holding it.

On Tuesday 4th October 1966 Basutoland acquired Self -Government (*Boipuso*). There were great celebrations through the country thereafter to be known officially as 'Lesotho'. We celebrated the day itself by walking to the top of the highest mountain, Maliphofu ('Mother of Wild Oxen'), above Ha Chooko, 8,900 feet above sea level. This was on foot and well worth the effort; and gave us an unrivalled view of our environs.

On the following day, we were invited to have lunch with Princess Marina at Marakabei on the banks of the Senqunyane, ten miles away. I was privileged to sit by the princess with the King , Moshoeshoe II, on her other side. She was so natural and approachable. She was keen to know just what we were doing in the middle of nowhere.

Our nurses were at little scared at being on duty at night and so we engaged a night watchman, Petrose who was supposed to do regular patrols of the hospital and call the doctor or more senior nurse when required. Petrose would come and knock on our bedroom window with his huge *knobkerrie* which was a sawn off branch of an Olive tree which he had enucleated. It resembled the weapon of giant ogres in the comics of childhood and I am sure he could have inflicted grievous bodily harm with the minimum of effort. Petrose was a tall formidable figure, with a skin and beard so black that he was quite invisible as he loomed up out of the dark. He insisted that I provide him with a large torch which consumed batteries at such an alarming rate that I suspected that he had a black market for them. It always amazed me just how fresh he looked in the morning after his hourly patrols in the night, which he assured me were punctiliously performed; but I had grave doubts as to whether he actually kept his night vigils conscientiously. One night I had been working late on clerical duties by Tilley Lamp (the Lister Engine having been put off some hours before) when I decided to go over to the hospital to check on a patient I was concerned about. As I approached the hospital kitchen I could see by the flickering light of a paraffin lamp a large form stretched out on the kitchen table, loudly snoring. I quietly went and saw my patient and as I walked back along the corridor I could hear the snoring of our night watchman reverberating through the quiet hospital. I marched around the kitchen but did not attempt to wake the slumbering Petrose. As a final gesture, I picked up his huge *knobkerrie* which was lying on top of the table beside him and locked it securely in my office till morning. Early next morning I invited Petrose to my office and confronted him with his prize knobkerrie lying on my desk. He was too shocked to say much as I handed him his dismissal notice. The irony of the situation made protracted explanations quite superfluous.

A far more efficient and effective night watchman proved to be a lovely Rhodesian Ridgeback dog we had bought on a shopping trip to Bloemfontein. We called him *Tau* (Lion) as these dogs were originally bred as lion hunters. I had built a kennel for Tau on our stoep and from there he could patrol the hospital grounds in search of tit bits from the staff who welcomed his visits and were not the least bit frightened of him, with his huge paws and amazing energy. The Basotho who did not know Tau were terrified of his speed and agility compared with their own emaciated and underfed creatures. As a young dog when tired of stripping washing skilfully from the washing line he would enthusiastically greet all visitors to the hospital. He would rush up to blanketed strangers and fasten his teeth on to the edge of their blankets, resolutely refusing to let go and prancing up and down in a frenzy of exuberant activity until eventually called of by a member of staff. This performance was a huge game which Tau enjoyed, and it had the merit of keeping away unwelcome intruders and advertised the arrival of unexpected patients most effectively.

In November 1966 we experienced a tremendous hail-storm. Hail stones the size of golf balls pelted down on the corrugated iron roofs and many staff and patients really thought it was the end of the world as a thatched rondavel roof tended to minimise such impact. Such hail-storms were not rare and we had been warned if out on horseback to dismount, remove the saddle and use it as a head shield. Lightning could also be quite frightening. One day Hazel drove the Land Rover to the Store and was only a few feet away from a lightning strike which made a deep gaping crack in the ground. Thank God for rubber tyres – she was only shocked.

The hospital was nearly always full and sometimes we had to improvise beds on the floor for the least ill patients – they didn't seem to mind.

We had lots of visitors before Christmas, who willingly lent a hand in laying floor tiles in the Nurse's Home, which was at last nearing completion. It had taken nine months, but we were very proud of our first DIY effort – not least Egbert who had put such personal care and hard work into this important addition to what we had called Phase II of the hospital.

In the New Year of 1967 feverish activity in equipping and furnishing the Nurse's Home culminated in the official opening on 12th January. The ceremony was performed by the Bishop of Springfield, Illinois in the United States of America, which was partnered with our own diocese. Bishop John drove Bishop Albert Chambers up to the hospital for a couple of days. Bishop

Chambers arrived in a black suit and chain-smoked cigarettes wherever he went. After taking two or three puffs at a cigarette, he then threw it down to the ground. John Maseli delighted in following him round like a personal body-guard and sedulously collected all the large episcopal stubs to smoke in his pipe.

The visiting Bishop had a pasty face like many Americans and wore a bright purple cassock and biretta when he discarded his black suit. He told me that he always dictated his correspondence as he drove around his diocese at home. This was in marked contrast to Bishop John who usually dressed informally, quietly smoked a pipe of pretty rough 'Horse-shoe' tobacco imported in little canvas bags for the Basotho, and wrote nearly all his own letters by hand to people in the diocese and to many supporters overseas. The Bishops shared a common faith but worked in such entirely different settings. I don't think either of them would have willingly exchanged jobs, but both were dedicated, holy men who worked equally hard in leading their very different peoples.

Early in February we had very heavy rains with seven inches of rain in three days. We heard that the Mantšonyane River was in full flood and no workers were able to cross to the hospital from Ha Chooko. We went down to investigate and found the river like a heavy sea with great waves that were in the process of washing away our beloved footbridge, which the schoolboys of St. Andrew's had erected. It was like witnessing a shipwreck with ropes and timbers being hurled into the fast flowing river never to be seen again. The bridge had taken four days to erect and was entirely destroyed in about four hours. It had been most useful over the two and a half years, in getting to and from Ha Chooko and was much mourned by the thousands who had used it to get to hospital and store. In some ways it was a warning to us, that building something is one thing, but making sure it survives is another. This made us more determined than ever to ensure as far as we possibly could that the hospital of St James which we had built, would not only continue its important work, but be capable of further development in serving the Basotho and expansion of its outreach into the remoter parts of the whole area of the central Maloti.

I made two or three abortive attempts to establish outstation clinics. There would be resident nurse to be visited from the hospital, at Lesobeng, Ha Mafa and Likalaneng, but for a variety of reasons, these plans never came to fruition, - not least was the time involved in visiting and liasing with these places and local difficulties in building by the local people.

In March, Dr. Michael Moore of the Flying Doctor Service visited us and enthused us with trying to build an airstrip close to the hospital. We were sure that this would prove a great help both with easier contact with Maseru and also with outlying clinics in the future.

At this time, Dorothy, our Matron decided to take her well earned retirement after working in Africa for more than a third of a century and as our first matron for more than three years. Dorothy brought to this work at St. James such a wealth of experience and organising ability and wonderful friendship and loyalty, that she was going to be difficult to replace. However, we fetched Grace Daintrey from Bloemfontein so that she could spend a little time with Dorothy before she left. This proved a good move in that Grace, a much younger and more agile woman, could gain some 'wrinkles' from the veteran before agreeing to take on the job herself. Dorothy had a fantastic send off by the staff with a feast and many parting gifts including a Basotho hat which suited her very well. Dorothy planned to set up home in Torquay with a friend but they eventually found Clevedon less expensive for retired missionaries.

Grace soon decided to stay and threw herself enthusiastically into consolidating Dorothy's work in her own way. She had gained quite a lot of experience in Botswana and Malawi and as a health visitor in the UK.

Our stalwart first Staff Nurse, Pauline was still with us and worked well with Mary Anne Molikoe. They were joined by a third Staff Nurse, Veronica Malibo, who was the daughter of a Mosotho Anglican priest in the lowlands. Our six Nurse Aids were busy preparing for the Home Nursing Certificate of the Lesotho Red Cross in 6 months time. Hazel took over duties as driver of the Land Rover Ambulance as well as wardenship of the Nurses' Home. She also managed to supervise the growing of vegetables for the hospital in spite of running our home and entertaining visitors.

We coped with a further epidemic of Typhoid Fever, which began in the autumn and reached its zenith in the following spring. The first case was in a village that I visited on horseback and had to spend the night on a mud floor. I brought back some fleas with me. They didn't seem to like the taste of me, but Hazel always suffered the most. This sometimes happened when I returned from the clinic at Marakabei. The problem was solved by getting patients to take off their blankets outside and give them a good shake, before entering the clinic!

Hazel accompanied me to Ha Leronti, a village about a mile away to investigate a severe outbreak of Typhoid. We lived the whole day on boiled eggs and brought several children back in the Land Rover Ambulance and treated dozens of older people at home with the wonder antibiotic, Chloromycetin. The spring in this village was on the main bridal path, so we took steps to get it properly protected and immunised those in the whole village who had not yet succumbed to the dreaded bug. At one stage, we had twenty-four children with typhoid in the hospital and had to top and tail them under strict barrier nursing. By June 1967 the operating theatre was equipped with a Japanese Operating table, which was put to good use for the usual assault cases and accident victims. We also did quite a number of skin grafts as the colder weather approached. We never had a case of appendicitis in a Mosotho in the area. I think it was due to the high roughage diet which people consumed.

In the midwifery department we delivered quite a number of delightful twins. We always managed to deal with the problem of obstructed labour using a simple Spanish technique called 'Zarate's Supra-pubic Symphisiotomy' which gave a 20% increase in pelvic outlet allowing sometimes for a normal delivery. From time to time a forceps delivery was required. The great benefit of this operation was that the pelvic outlet was permanently enlarged so that the next confinement was provided for, as many mothers might not be able to reach the hospital at some future date.

We had two cases of fatal liver failure in one day, which I strongly suspected as being due to taking of toxic doses of herbal remedies. This was unusual as most of the traditional herbalists had a vast and accurate knowledge of herbs, which they used to good effect in treating many maladies. I became very friendly with one traditional herbal doctor (Ngaka Chitja), called `Mafanti. She confided in me a number of remedies which had been passed on to her. She even offered me a particular root, which I could administer to my wife to ensure that she remained faithful to me!

We had a gang of men working hard to make an airstrip, which ran the length of the hospital grounds in front of the hospital. It was only half completed in mid September when Dr. Michael Moore flew low over us as if he were trying to land. Egbert with his usual quick thinking and agility quickly ran and removed the fence at the south end of the grounds to enable the first landing to take place. Dozens of people seemed to appear from nowhere to witness at close quarters this historic moment. The airstrip was completed by the end of November ready for emergency use without having to take down the fence!

At this time we had forty-five patients in the hospital but still only officially had thirty-five beds.

One day in early summer there was a great commotion in the valley with young men dancing, shouting and gathering firewood. It was the beginning of an Initiation (Circumcision) School. They soon disappeared into the remoter mountains for the secret rites of the initiation.

In December we installed a new and more powerful engine for lighting purposes. On Christmas Eve we walked over to Ha Chooko for Midnight Mass. On return there was a lady with a miscarriage requiring surgery and so I retired to bed at 4am on Christmas morning. We had a delightful carol service in the hospital later in the morning. We had many visitors staying with us for what was to be our last Christmas at the hospital.

Early in January Dr. James Maxwell Jones and his wife, Hilda, visited us and agreed to come and replace us. It was not an easy decision to leave St James' Hospital, but after seven years of working in such an isolated spot we felt it was right to return to the U.K before becoming 'Mountain Happy'. We had seen this happen to priests, teachers, traders and others who had stayed too long in the mountains. We were determined to heed the early signs and symptoms of this malady. It was time to hand over a functioning unit to others with new and different gifts. We had accomplished a task which many had forecast as impossible in such a remote location with difficult terrain and climate.

Since 1961 we had treated over 25,000 out-patients: this was also the estimated total population of the area we served. In four years over 1,300 patients had stayed in the hospital and more than 350 babies had been born there. The average daily number staying in the hospital had doubled in the last two years.

We had given a lot to the people of Mantšonyane, but had received far more than we were ever able to give (more about this later). Before we left we were given many gifts including two mohair rugs made to last forever and two Basotho blankets which we were made to wear as honorary Basotho. Pauline as the longest serving nurse said some kind and touching words. When I replied I said: 'We are going home but our hearts will stay right here in the Maloti mountains'. As we left and drove round the bend in the track we glanced back at 'our baby' we had helped to 'conceive' and 'bring to birth'. We thanked God for the privilege of being allowed to do this and for the multitude of people who had helped us in so many ways – we had just been the initial ground troops. We were confident that God would send the necessary re-enforcements in the years ahead.

PART TWO

'A foundation on which others have built'. (I Cor 3.10a CEV)

The history of St. James' hospital so far has been an expanded personal diary of the first seven years.

Part Two of this account covers subsequent developments over the past thirty- three years during which more than twenty doctors have carried the work forward and extended it up to the present time. It has been like completing a huge jig-saw puzzle from which some pieces have been difficult to find and others have so far not been located. Multiple sources of information have been used to produce as full an account as possible, including personal accounts provided by many of those who have served the hospital over the years; some written at the time, others kindly sent to me recently.

Chapter 5. UNEXPECTED HELP.

Dr. James Maxwell Jones, who had worked at Bethnal Green Medical Mission in London, was only able to serve for about six months in 1968 owing to his wife's serious illness. His expertise as a surgeon was sadly of only temporary benefit and was cut short just at the time when it would have been most useful and so the hospital was without a resident doctor for about a year. John Swift assisted as general maintenance officer and was kept busy transporting patients to the Q.E.II Hospital in Maseru when they could not be adequately cared for locally.

Grace Daintrey, the second matron, coped very well during this 'doctor-less time', but unfortunately had to return to the UK to nurse her very elderly sick father. She was replaced by Judy Moore until Anne Woolman was appointed fourth matron and coped very valiantly without a doctor for about a year. She had no hesitation in going out on horseback to investigate and treat epidemics of typhoid fever in the villages.

Father David Wells, an Australian member of the Society of the Sacred Mission, was appointed by the bishop to act as administrator in the absence of a medical superintendent, in addition to his duties as Rector of the parish of St. James' with all its outstations. Father David was a trained accountant and had worked in Papua New Guinea. Donations towards the hospital maintenance fell sharply and so a special appeal was launched to remedy the situation. The staff at this time was headed by Anne Woolman as matron, who was assisted by the faithful Sister Pauline, four Staff Nurses, four Nurse Aids, and eight domestics. John Swift as maintenance officer was ably assisted by four local Basotho, headed by Egbert Monese, who had amply proved his worth and was, together with Pauline Sixishe, a continuous source of stability and local knowledge, enabling the hospital to survive quite a difficult period.

By the end of January 1969, patient attendance had begun to increase steadily and the number of in-patients reached an all time peak since the hospital had opened six years before. This was remarkable without a resident doctor and a tribute to the marvellous teamwork led by Anne and Father David. It was however a great relief to the staff, when, rather unexpectedly, USPG sent a Jewish doctor, Nicholas Cohen, to take charge of a Christian Mission Hospital! (God works in mysterious ways his wonders to perform) Nicholas arrived on the 1st May 1969 on a two year-contract as Medical Superintendent. He came at the right time and threw himself wholeheartedly into the work and identified closely with the Basotho throughout his time in the Maloti.

Nicholas was a Cambridge graduate who had gained a double MRCP (Edinburgh & London) He had worked at the famous Guy's Hospital in London. He and Thérèse soon settled at St James'.

After his first six months at the helm Nicholas wrote:

I am just beginning to understand the Basotho and their way of life. The strangeness of coming here from the greyness and the crowd of London has changed to a sense of feeling that in one way it is home.

His friendliness and rapport with the Basotho was much appreciated and twenty-eight years later he was still being asked about by old patients!

Nicholas describes his first experiences of working at Mantšonyane:

The winter was quite mild with snow on a few occasions and the wards were not too full; but now with the start of summer we have today several patients sleeping on the floor. Nearly all the children are underfed and, though many have infections such as pneumonia N and measles, the lack of food and the wrong type of food are the greatest problem. We have therefore restarted the Under-fives Clinic. We have converted the laundry to use for this purpose and are going to build a new laundry. We hope that the mothers will come every month to get food, injections, and education in simple hygiene. The teaching of the mother is really most important, the food being used as bait. All are very enthusiastic, but not all are willing to pay the charge of two shillings a month which is sometimes beyond their resources.

We continue to see patients at the Government Health Centre at Ha Marakabei every week. Often there are no other drugs available than Aspirin, Vitamins, and a sort of local "Alka-Seltzer" mixture. There is little opportunity to display great medical treatment in such circumstances! Our own clinics, however, are well equipped with drugs sent by mule from the hospital. Only about twenty patients attend these clinics each visit but we are trying to be patient till they are better known. Most Basotho still go to their own traditional doctor before consulting us.

John Swift left the hospital after finishing the new airstrip, thus completing nine months service to the hospital during difficult times.

Nicholas reported further:

We are visiting two clinics, Ha Mafa, two hours ride away, and Ha Khomari, Lesobeng but the people are incredibly slow to do anything. Ha Khomari seems a better prospect—I saw many people on my first visit and there is a reasonable site for a permanent building which could serve most of the Lesobeng valley.

In June 1970 Nicholas commented further;

Delay in British Aid (£2M a year) has hit all sections of the people hard – but hardest of course the poorest. The hospital grant from the government has been reduced by another 10% so we only receive £1125 p.a. in all.

It has not rained seriously since 16th January. It is early winter and light snow has fallen on the mountains but not enough to soak through the outer crust. There's a strong cold wind blowing though the sun has been warm during the middle of the day. The gusts blow up dust storms, which swirl about you on horseback like riding through the desert. The

Mantšonyane River is just a series of pools. Many of the springs in the villages have dried completely and people are walking from one place near here about an hour to get water. The hospital spring still runs but it is only producing about 15 gallons per hour. As a result of the drought, the maize crop has failed all over. It looks grim for the people and the sheep when we get round to spring and there's nothing to eat. We can't expect rain until October and the only hope is for good snow.

We are running at about the maximum capacity of thirty-five beds. A very sick little boy with Measles and Pneumonia came in yesterday. He'd not had enough to eat for months and his face has pealed markedly as it often does in Africans. He's lying in a makeshift steam-tent constructed out of sheets and a Ronald Searle-like contraption of an old oil drum with a length of tubing heating on a blue flame heater that John Swift had cleverly put together. His mother brought him to the rondavel clinic at Ha Mafa and then carried him for three hours on her back to the hospital.

Perhaps the most remarkable and lucky woman also comes from Ha Mafa. Mother of ten, she went into labour in her hut and started to push too early. Her womb ruptured and the baby was forced into the abdominal cavity, together with a lot of blood. She would have been in terrible pain but managed to walk here! Most women would have been dead inside an hour. In my absence Anne radioed the flying doctor who happened to be at the airfield with a plane at hand. Anne got the steriliser going and the nurses scrubbed up, so that when the doctor arrived he walked straight into the theatre. Thanks to the people of Dunchurch Rural Deanery who had made the radio possible, the mother was well and up only eight hours later.

Anne went on a well-earned holiday for a month and Carole Willan took her place. She had been here for a few weeks already, 'learning the trade'. Great news is that Peter Beresford has arrived from the U.K. last week, full of enthusiasm to maintain the buildings and proceed with the new projects. Most important of all the staff news is that Mrs Pauline Maema, who may be the best Mosotho nurse in the country, has come to St. James' Hospital.

Nicholas reported in the Nursing Mirror. About riding to Thaba Tseka Hospital (Paray) in the snow:

I was covering both hospitals at the time and we got caught in a blizzard. I remember eating roast mealies (maize) with some herd-boys in a field. They were also roasting field mice but I declined to share in the feast.

Nicholas Cohen has also kindly provided a recent account of his memories of this period for inclusion in this book,

Ha Mafa Clinic was just one very ordinary rondavel. We waited for months to get straw on the roof. I sent a tin trunk of medicines there by mule and visited twice a month on horseback. Once a month I would go to Lesobeng by horse over a wild and lonely pass, which cut across to the Methalaneng Valley. This route was so steep and rocky that one had to climb alongside the horse.

For a tooth extraction I would often take a chicken instead of money payment. Going back to the hospital I would put two chickens in the saddlebags either side and head home for dinner but they were very tough.

Ha Khomari Clinic, Lesobeng was opened at the top of the valley in the shadow of Thaba Moea because it was mot accessible from Methalaneng. Still it took 5-6 hours on horseback from Ha Mafa. Often the Ha Mafa Clinic extended into the afternoon and I arrived after dark at Ha Khomari. One day there was a wonderful plant growing outside the clinic. I asked what it was — Marijuana of course. We were very innocent in those days.

In August 1970 Nicholas was able to write:

We now have four clinics being visited Ha Mafa, Likalaneng, Marakabei and Ha Khomari, Lesobeng with more patients than ever before and more deliveries already than in the whole of last year.

We are very happy here. It is a good life and the isolation does not worry us. Friends visit from Maseru and there is quite an international set working for the relief agencies. The staff are good people and there is a friendly atmosphere. Egbert of course bears most of the weight on his shoulders for practical problems. Our two new 10000-gallon tanks should soon allow us to have spray irrigation, which should increase vegetable yields. We now have three horses, which are worked quite hard.

On 5th December 1970 the British Medical Journal published a delightful article entitled, 'Personal View', by Nicholas:

I am the only doctor here but I say it with no disrespect to my traditional colleagues who have been in the field a lot longer than I have and are better psychologists than most; it's just that we work along different lines.

Basotho ponies are good climbers over the rock faces, over which the bridle paths wander, but progress is slow and if you want to use your energy in a better way than wearing out your backside, then preventive medicine is an attractive alternative. The hospital is young, having only been here 8years, so ideas of prevention are still fresh to the people who think in terms of dramatic cures; but we do have four out- clinics visited regularly, a flourishing ante-natal clinic which can provide Caesarean Section under local anaesthetic if they get into trouble at the end of the run and an Under-fives Clinic which is popular.

Egbert Monese is our maintenance man. His hair is greying and every day he reads the lesson at the chapel prayers in Sesotho, picking his way through the occasional tangle of Roman names with respect, wearing a bulky raincoat more suited to a coxswain of a lifeboat. His greeting is invariably warm and he exits backwards from your presence or skips along to open a door before you. The hospital is his home and he works all hours seven days a week. He is the local capitalist. Several daughters have been exchanged for cattle successfully and he rents out his oxen to plough like Mr. Hertz.

On one occasion we had been drying cabbage from the garden, and getting suspicious asked Egbert if he stopped to wash the vegetables. He had not. What about the worms, Egbert? I can still see them lying with the leaves. 'Never mind those, doctor. They'll dry the same as the rest. And they did.

One day I was operating with our relief matron from Pondoland. All was going well when the patient woke up. With the snow outside, the operating theatre was so cold that the ether was failing to vaporise properly. 'When I was in Pondoland, we used nitrous oxide', matron began. I cut her short. 'When I was at Guy's Hospital we opened hearts and put in new valves and the anaesthetist put catheters in the radial arteries and intubated patients'. She was not impressed. 'When I was in Pondoland we operated four days a week', was her retort!

Here are some recent memories recently recalled by Nicholas:

Our daughter, Natasha was born in December 1970 right in the middle of summer in the Southern Hemisphere. Thérèse drove down alone at night to where I was sleeping at Likalaneng on the way to Maseru to say she could be starting labour. It was a long way in the blackness. Next morning she had stopped labour but it was snowing! The snow became so deep that Jim Conway, the Irish doctor, who was due to come from Thaba Tseka for the delivery could not make it. No way either for a plane because the clouds were too low. The next evening Thérèse went seriously into labour. I remember passing the garden where the tomato plants were covered in snow. She stayed at home until the middle of the night. Then she came to the labour room where a Mosotho was giving birth. We put on classic guitar music by Segovia, which I brought from the house. The labour went fine until the end. She was tired and there was some delay. Finally, and not wanting to do so, I used a vacuum extractor to deliver a really fat and later pink baby girl. She was born in a caul and I could not see her face. I remember a feeling of shock but matron just said, ' Take off the membranes'. Natasha weighed 9.7 pounds - a record I think for the hospital and certainly the first European baby born there. I carried her outside into the corridor in my arms and the staff waiting immediately said 'It is `Malehloa (Mother of the snow)', which remained her official second name.

I had a bucket of water poured over me the traditional way of announcing the birth of a baby girl! 'Malehloa was on horseback, Basotho style by the age of six weeks, wrapped in a blanket on her mother's back. Before the age of two months she spent her first night in a rondavel in a village and had been put to suckle at the breast of a Mosotho woman.

A month after 'Malehloa's birth, we had a huge party with eight sheep to be eaten and lots of mabele (millet) beer. It was a real Basotho Pitiki (Food given to women who have helped at a confinement) with dancing and chanting and we roasted the sheep outside. Hundreds of people came to see the strange baby of Ntate Ngaka. The hills were black with people moving from all directions. I wore a Russian peasant style shirt with a Russian black fur hat and Thérèse dressed up in Xhosa beads while holding the baby. We certainly looked weird when I now see the picture.

There was a tragic side to the unseasonable snowstorm. A plane from Semonkong crashed at the top of the last pass but it took several days to locate it. The pilot had risked flying through cloud and missed clearing the peak by a few metres.

Our completed airstrip was rather fine, smooth gravel over the rock surface and quite wide. The problems were the planes could only land and take off in one direction because the valley was so narrow. After 11.0 a.m. flights were often impossible because of crosswinds. The runway was also at two levels with a step in the middle to a higher plateau, which meant that one could not see the end from the front of the hospital. There were not many planes, but sometimes I took my role as an airport director quite seriously. When we heard a plane, for example, I would leave the clinic and, still in my white coat, stand with my small fire extinguisher near the runway. A useless procedure but it kept me occupied. We never had an accident. One day the plane came but instead of landing flew very low over our heads. This was repeated several times and so I ran up to the invisible start of the airstrip and found a herd-boy calmly grazing his donkey right on the normal landing point. The pilot was furious on landing and I had a job persuading him that from the ground we could see nothing of the end of the airstrip.

Regularly the water pump would break down and we would have no water for the hospital. You could run a hospital without electricity but not without water. Oxfam provided money for two 10,000 gallon tanks to be erected above the hospital grounds next to sister Pauline's house. The idea was to pump up water to the tanks as a reserve supply to feed the hospital if the pump broke down. Seeing 'Me Pauline walk down from her house, with her imposing figure, was always a good start to the day. With Oxfam support and about 100 workers (women as well as men), a trench was dug and the reservoirs erected. 'Me Pauline had a special pipe supply for her house. The hospital benefited also from this project.

I only had experience as a student and 3 months as a house surgeon before coming to St, James'. I brought an Oxford EMO machine with me and, for larger surgery, used ether with a halothene induction.

Operations on smashed skulls were rather common. I learned how to trephine and raised bone flaps. We had some great results with people speaking again and using limbs. At first Thérèse used to read to me from Hamilton Bailey's Emergency Surgery, which we took into the operating theatre.

Dr Anthony Barker at Nqutu in Zululand showed me his method of doing Caesarean sections under local anaesthetic. My first operation was for a woman with obstructed labour due to transverse lie. All went well but the baby was hydrocephalic but we had saved the mother's life. She was the chief's daughter and so St. James' reputation went high and Morena Toka was delighted. I did about 12 Caesarean sections in all and all did well.

Nicholas reflected further on his time at the hospital in his B.M.J. article:

So what was it that brings one to a place like this? Or to put it in another way, what is it that keeps one in such a place? Being a Jew, it is not the missionary side. And anyway the Basotho have troubles enough of their own without the added burden of Judaism- that would be too unkind. Also it is not the self-destructive urge to throw away one's career, as some kind friends have hinted, but rather the chance to develop different skills and to use one's creativity in a challenging field where one can get really close and try to become part of the people one is trying to help.

[I would suggest that this is missionary activity of great value. The Sesotho for missionary is 'moruti har'a lichaba', which means ' teacher amongst the people.' Nicholas was certainly that! - Editor.]

Nicholas continues;

Only four doctors have visited me in the past 18 months and I miss the professional contact and the sharper critical standards that come with it. After the in-fighting and reference quoting of a professorial ward round, it is a little soft to go it alone. But Africa gets into your blood and a day in the laboratory seems tame in comparison to wakening in a village hut at dawn on a goat skin mattress. The work is not always as exciting as it seems from afar; there is a routine and therefore times of frustration and despair. Too many people want too much from you at the same time and your spirit cannot take it. Schweitzer has put it clearly: 'There are not a great number of diseases, but required is a great amount of patience which I have not got.' I can now see what he means!

In April 1971 Nicholas Cohen returned to the UK to pursue his research career in London. During his two years St. James' he helped to develop and extend the work of the hospital and was much loved by the Basotho, although he did not always see eye to with Father David and the Bishop. His contribution as a son of Israel was as significant as it was unexpected and he was not far from 'the kingdom of God'! Notably he was the first doctor to perform abdominal surgery, to establish firmly the outstation clinics and lay good foundations for the development of a Primary Health Care Programme.

After Nicholas's departure the hospital was once more without a resident doctor, but was visited by the flying doctor twice a month and had radio contact with him three times a day.

Edgar Gapper had recently been appointed as Maintenance Officer. He was no stranger to Mantšonyane having served as a lay brother of SSM at Ha Chooko for five years. As Brother William he was well known to the local Basotho. He reported that the Land-Rover ambulance was on its last legs. There was a Ford Ranchero that was a struggle to drive in bad weather and was getting damaged underneath. Anne hated driving it even in good weather. The new laundry was progressing well and was to include a sewing and ironing room. The new airstrip meant that Egbert's little house and the potato store had to be moved. At this time efforts were being made to finance a new maternity block. Egbert Monese, John Maseli, and Jacote Thene soldiered on together with a fourth man called Thabo. The old water pump finally gave up the ghost and so a much more powerful centrifugal pump was purchased. There were eventual plans to have two complete units.

Anne Woolman continued splendid work as Matron without a resident doctor. She could not refuse a request for a new clinic at Ha Khotso (five hours ride away) when the chief sent horses and a guide and also provided a rondavel for the clinic.

Anne saved one life by successfully performing a major operation-something she had never done before – under instruction over the radio from a doctor in Maseru, with a nurse holding a book of instructions in front of her, while she did the job. Afterwards she was regarded as a doctor by the local people.

In May 1971 Anne went on a very well earned furlough, Judy Moore taking her place while she was away. Judy had acted as Matron before. She had originally come from the U.K. to work under a voluntary service organisation. As there was insufficient work to occupy her she happily transferred to St. James'. She later married Mr. Clarke, the local storekeeper.

Mrs Jean Ashton, a delightful and charming Australian lady, came to work at the hospital for some time. She looked after the kitchen, housekeeping and performed a great deal of administrative duties, including the accounts. Anne Woolman returned to duty in January 1972 but Judy gladly stayed on to help.

In the spring of 1972 Sister Tessa of the Community of the Holy Name, Leribe, in the lowlands, visited the hospital. She found Anne busy cleaning up the wounds of a man who had been beaten severely for stealing wheat- an eye opener for Sister Tessa. In the autumn she returned with three Basotho sisters and stayed for three months, giving much needed nursing assistance to Anne while the Basotho sisters did much valuable pastoral visiting, both in the hospital and the local villages. Such visits from the CHN sisters became an established pattern over the next few years. The sisters' visits were so much appreciated by the local Basotho and one of them worked as a Nurse Aid in the hospital. Sister Tessa enabled Anne to have a break from time to time.

In January 1973, after a year and nine months without a resident doctor at St. James', Dr. Brian King and his wife, Siân, an Anglican couple, were at last sent by USPG from the UK. This gave a new impetus to the work at the hospital, which had miraculously survived without a doctor. Wonderful devotion by the staff as well as help from outside had made this possible. Laus Deo!

Chapter 6 : CONSOLIDATION OF CONFIDENCE

Dr Brian King and his wife Siân contribute their experience from January 1973 to December 1974.

We were, you might say, guided by an unseen hand; drawn inexorably; called, even. Siân and I knew that Mantšonyane was for us. It started when we approached USPG to ask about medical posts in their Missions in Africa. They said, yes, they were in need of a doctor in a small mountainous country in the southern tip of Africa. They said, 'It so happens that the Matron from the hospital is on furlough, and would you like to meet her?'. We met Anne Woolman; she seduced us with descriptions of a small but thriving hospital in the middle of nowhere, and she enticed us with photos. Soon after, USPG said 'It so happens that the priest from the Mission is also here in London'. We met Father David, and we knew then we were destined for Mantšonyane. USPG said, 'Would you like to meet the Bishop? He's on leave just now'. We met Bishop John Maund but by that time we were well and truly called.

The Hospital had by now been over a year without a doctor. I was keen to know what sort of medicine I would be able to practice, out there on my own and so recently out of Medical School. Was I kidding myself I could cope? I got in touch with Nick Cohen, we met up, we talked African Hospital medicine. I knew then that I would be able to manage. Yes, there would be testing times; yes, I could forget a lot of what I had been taught about high-tech Medicine; yes, I would have to be prepared to improvise, to do my best, however humble or ineffectual, to be able to face failure as well as triumph. I took his advice and did some training in Orthopaedics and Trauma; spent some time with an Anaesthetics consultant who had spent many years in the wilder parts of India; attended the Dental School in Leicester Square and learned to pull teeth. Also, we agreed to spend the first three months of our two-year stint, at the Scott Hospital in Morija, in the lowlands of Lesotho. There, we came under the joyful influence of Ted and Ilse Germond, and I learned many more 'tricks of the trade' as well as picking up the basics of Sesotho, the language of the whole country.

Someone visiting the hospital at that time, might have found him or herself in the midst of a ready-made community with a cast of many.

Dramatis Personæ:

Brian King, Greenhorn doctor if ever there was one; bit of a Jack of All Trades, and prepared to tackle most things,

Sian King, 'Mother' of all Trades; book-keeper, ambulance driver, you name it, she did it,

Rosalind Ferguson, Adding glamour to the usual role of Matron, hospital lynchpin; nurse, midwife, tutor, confidante for the staff, artist in residence,

Father David, Australian priest, accountant, horseman, beer-drinker, endless supply of aisle-rolling Oz jokes,

Sr. Pauline Sixishe, Powerful woman and much respected in the community; a fund of local knowledge, not to be crossed; but with a ready twinkle in her eye and eager to see the humorous side of events,

Ntate Egbert, Senior member of the 'Men' who looked after the Hospital and did the heavy work,

John and Judy Clarke, ran the nearby store, agents for Collier & Yeats who supplied most of our needs at the Hospital, including fresh milk from their cow and legs of pork smoked in their back yard,

Jean Ashton, Elderly Australian general helps-person; secretary, companion for Thabo the Dog,.

Bishop John Maund, Widely loved and respected in the Mountains of Lesotho, travelled everywhere on horseback,

William Gapper, Originally one of the Brothers at the Mission, left to marry one of the nurses; general supervisor and mechanic,

Jack, Took over from William, cherished the simple life of the Basotho, but they wanted him to stay on our side of the line....

Various nurses, nurse-aids, men, cooks; *Ntate* Night-Watchman; visiting travellers, students, anthropologists, priests, and a selection of 'permanent' patients, usually small unclaimed children; cats, dogs.

When we arrived, the hospital was generally in good shape; but a number of clinics had been allowed to run down, and needed to be re-opened. Before long we were operating out-posts at Ha Khomari, Likalaneng, and Marakabei. The monthly clinic at Ha Khomari was always a rather special trip for Sian and myself - it was a six hour ride on horse-back, accompanied by a nurse or two, a dispenser, and pack-mules laden with equipment, medicines and clothes. The clinic was held the following day crammed into a small rondavel; at night we laid out our sleeping bags and slept, exhausted; and on the third day we rode home to the undoubted comfort of a hot bath and a soft bed.

The hardships, and stoicism of the people were amply illustrated when, one afternoon, I noticed a group of men leading in a horse. On its back was a boy of fifteen, looking a bit pale but nevertheless holding his head up and betraying no pain. He was tied, I soon noticed, so that he would not fall off. As the men untied him they explained that two days previously he had fallen into a gully and broken his leg. He had been brought across the mountains to the hospital for us to mend him

Luckily we had all the right equipment; he was soon in a hospital bed, awaiting the skills of the European doctor who knew how to do anything. I, for my part, was deep in a book of Orthopaedics, how to fix fractured legs! I had learned all this sort of thing at Medical School, but never done it. I set to work, hammering a stainless steel pin through his shin bone (under anaesthetic - I'm not that heartless), attached him to some weights and pulleys. It never ceased to amaze me what variety of useful bits of equipment were stored away in cupboards there. Lo and behold, his leg mended perfectly; a few weeks later he was up and about, and in due course, the same group of men came to collect him and take him home

Things didn't go right every time. How could we expect them to? We hadn't the facilities, the skills, the knowledge or the confidence to make a success of every illness, accident or emergency that came our way. But would we cope? How would we deal with disaster? I was to find out the hard way one afternoon, when Sister Sixishe called me to say that one of the Bakhachane (pregnant mothers) was in labour and having problems breathing. My heart sank - it was the woman with the heart valve disease, who had had a stormy passage through previous labours. She had declined an offer to send her to the Hospital in the lowlands. Now, the strain of labour was getting the better of her heart. Her lungs were filling with oedema fluid and she was literally drowning as she lay on the labour couch. Inside me, I was dumbstruck. Outwardly, I followed theory and instinct and gave her the drugs that might save her. They didn't work on her. Her labour weakened, and so did her heart. We watched, horrified. The nurses comforted her as she slipped into unconsciousness. They listened for the baby's heart - it, too, was failing. Should we do a Caesarean and save the baby? It would kill the mother, that was for sure, but she was doomed anyway. But could I put a scalpel into a living person, no time for the niceties of anaesthesia? Time seemed to play with us - it went too fast so I had no time to think straight, make a plan - it went too slow, I wanted this thing over and done with.

Finally, I steeled myself and performed, in effect, a post-mortem Caesarean. The baby was dead. I was in shock, numbed. Medical School training never mentioned this sort of thing. I needed to think. Was this a blunder too far? Was this a signal to bail out? I made my way to the peace and the quiet of the chapel. God was waiting for me. I thought, many years later, how an episode like this, back home, would have sent me scuttling for the phone and my lawyer. I wept for the mother and I wept for the child. And I knew then that God would send his comfort and his support to each of us, and that we would do our best to return His love by continuing with our work.

Siân writes:

My role at Mantšonyane was 'doctor's wife' - this much was made clear from the start by USPG. The idea of a happily married committed couple was very important and, although I was not paid, I was expected to make a substantial contribution to the work of the hospital in whatever capacity I could. By profession I am a librarian, which may, at first, seem a less than useful qualification; on my side, however, was youth (I was 24), a great enthusiasm for the work of the hospital, and a long-awaiting fulfilment to work in a developing country. As it turned out, there were many responsibilities that I was able to take on, and I ended up working full-time on the numerous non-medical tasks that were essential to keep the place going.

To give some sort of idea of the variety of this work, it included:all the paperwork such as double-entry book-keeping (expertly trained by accountant Father David), rendering endless statistics to the Lesotho Ministry of Health, answering letters and begging for money, producing a Newsletter, paying all the staff, supervising and distributing all the food for the in-patients, which including deciding on the menu each day and keeping the huge amount of donated food under lock and key, driving the land-rover ambulance across almost non-existent mountain tracks to collect sick patients doing a radio-call twice a day to the flying doctor's base in Maseru, and requesting the plane when necessary to pick up seriously ill patients (there was no telephone) monitoring and ordering all the supplies such as fuel for the generator and drugs accompanying the medical staff (usually on horseback) to clinics, vaccination campaigns etc. where I would check in patients, give out drugs and generally lend moral support entertaining the huge number of visitors who would turn up without warning ranging from various Government officials, to anthropologists, tourists and fellow-Christians helping, when asked, in the pharmacy, the delivery room, the operating theatre, (mainly to swat the flies), the wards, the children's' clinic…

As is apparent from the above list, an ability to turn one's hand to anything, willingly, was perhaps the primary requirement for life at this remote outpost…and, of course, a huge sense of humour as well as a healthy respect for the Basotho people and their culture.

An illustration of this may be found in one of the more challenging jobs that fell to me - finding meat for the patients:

First, choose your sheep.

'Going to the butcher' in the mountains of Lesotho is a somewhat novel experience for someone straight from England. To start with, a sheep must be summoned, or rather a flock of sheep from which to choose.

'Ntate Egbert', I say to the foreman, 'we would like sheep this week, Can you find some for us?'

'Yes, mother - of course, mother - I will shout for them mother', he replies, setting off to shout across the mountain valley to a neighbouring village. I return to my typing and paperwork, calculating salaries, collecting fees and selling stamps until Ntate Egbert appears at my door, knocking cautiously.

'The sheep are here, mother!' I gratefully leave the paperwork for the warm sunshine outside and ponder the sheep…we have all the time in the world. It is a small flock, accompanied by their owner, our customary sheep-seller, but a bit of a crook into the bargain. The sheep are a mixed bunch - some quite woolly, others newly shorn with a few mohair goats as well. The sheep-seller, Ntate Mashapa, greets me like a long-lost friend and grins widely while we size each other up. It is Christmas, and we want four animals for a large feast for patients and staff.

'Which ones for sale, Ntate Mashapa'? I ask, in my stumbling Sesotho.

'Two sheep there...the one with the clipped ear, and the other one by the goat - and the two goats are also available'.

I gaze thoughtfully at the beasts in question. I have no idea how to tell a good sheep from a bad - I've never really even looked at a sheep before. They keep trying to escape from the circle we have automatically formed around them. The herd-boy, aged about eight, whistles expertly at them, and waves his stick. I have been told that 'it's all in the tail' - if it is fat, then the meat is good. If there is much wool, you have to look closely and feel the rump. I do so cautiously, and whisper to Ntate Egbert,

'How are they?'

'They are alright, mother', he replies, with a nervous glance towards Ntate Mashapa.

'How much?'

Ntate Mashapa grins, 'Two sheep there, and two goats, all for 36 Rand! I laugh openly,

'Nine Rand each! - I can do arithmetic too! - I'll have the four for 30 Rand'

'32 Rand?'

'OK by me' I finally responded. I was aware that he would still make a very good profit, but at least I had made a gesture towards bargaining, and I did rather fancy a goat skin for a bedside rug.

We shook hands on conclusion of the deal, after which I fetched the money while Ntate Mashapa, with a glint in his eye, produced a bill of sale as proof of ownership. I do not know how he acquires these, nor wish to know - what matters is that we go through the motions and everyone seems happy.

I then declare, with more confidence than I feel, 'We'll have two now, and two next week. The hospital workmen gather round to try and catch the beasts - two will be killed, and the other two will be daubed with paint to establish our ownership, then allowed to graze until needed. The killing is performed quickly, well out of my sight; the carcass is butchered for the patients' main meal, the liver reserved for the 'high protein' diets, the other offal for the staff and the head for the man who performed the slaughter - even here at the hospital we can retain this tradition.

The Christmas feast is a grand one - two pots full of meat boiling over open fires, whilst vegetables and 'papa' (the staple maize-based food) is prepared in the hospital kitchen. When the meat is cooked, the water is drained out and some precious oil added for a last minute fry - the result is delicious, and all are replete.

I step into the kitchen with the dirty dishes, and the sheep's head looks at me from a shelf - I turn away from its accusing eyes, and hope someone will eat it soon. The cooks laugh at my squeamishness, but I think they understand.

Brian continues:

By the time we were into our second year we had come to know many of the other 'mission' doctors in Lesotho. There was a feeling among all of us that we could, and should, co-operate in our efforts to improve the health services to the people. Thus was born the Private Hospitals Association of Lesotho (PHAL). We agreed to share the benefits of the donated equipment and supplies arriving regularly from around the world. We met to discuss clinical matters. We exchanged ideas, experiences and moral support.

How did we see the hospital develop, during our time there? Perhaps we saw the purpose, the context of the Mission Hospital become a little clearer. It had been started with a very clear and sincere vision - why it was there, what its philosophy was, how it sat in relation the Mission. During Nick Cohen's tenure, these 'givens' had been questioned - rightly so, because African hospital medicine generally was coming under scrutiny, and having to justify itself as well as accept new and unorthodox methodologies. Was it cost-effective? Was it bringing the right kind of 'medicine' to these isolated people? Was it spreading the right messages about health and progress? Nick Cohen had strong views and he did his best to abolish the use of bottle-feeding and advocated natural feeding, accompanied by regular child-care and developmental surveillance. He promoted vaccination campaigns and clinics. All of these I inherited; and we felt, as our time went by, that we were helping to consolidate, rather than innovate. We promoted the new teaching. We had, it is true, to maintain the confidence of the people there, by 'curing disease' and wielding the magic scalpel. But having done that, we re-iterated the message of Prevention by all possible means as the key to better health. And it was this, coupled with a determination to keep the hospital afloat financially, that won us the confidence of the Hospital Board, the committee in Maseru, chaired by the Bishop, whose responsibility it was to oversee the running and the success of the hospital.

Rosalind Sellers (Nee Ferguson) who was matron from December 1972 to March 1976 concludes this chapter:

While on a mission in Transkei, (where I was being introduced to some skills not included in the General Nurse training in the UK, and waiting for a permit to go to St Mary's Hospital, Ovamboland), I visited Lesotho and felt a tremendous exhilaration: it was relaxed, vibrant and stunningly beautiful. The glimpse was put aside as I was going elsewhere. Imagine my excitement when USPG asked me to go and help Anne Woolman in Mantšonyane while I was waiting for news of the permit. After an initial visit and a six week stint in a Language school I returned, to be told that if I wanted to stay I would have to be matron! Anne had left, the senior nurse, 'Me Pauline Sixishe had no desire to be matron, and there wasn't anyone else. In great trepidation, I accepted a three month trial, thinking that that would be that! After all, I was twenty-four and had not even been in charge of a ward. There must have been tremendous support from all around or it would have been totally impossible.

One of the nurse assistants told me that it would take people at least a year and a half to accept me, so patience was to be a vital ingredient. Time after time I felt totally inadequate for what came up, and was often aware of help. The job included looking after the nurses, visiting outstations, helping with outpatients, (including taking X-rays, sometimes setting simple fractures, suturing, or doing dental extractions), being responsible for theatre, promoting health education, any general help around that was needed, and trying to stand in for the doctor in his absence. I was also expected to sort out personal problems, some of which were embedded in the Basotho culture, and far beyond my capability to resolve. Happily the people appeared to be very accepting and did not seem to blame us as much when things did not work out well.

THE NURSES.

Sister Pauline Sixishe had been there since the hospital started. She had six children, mostly grown up and married, all of whom she entirely supported through high school. (Her oldest son, Desmond became private secretary to Prime Minister Jonathan.) She had worked in Cape Town, (Children's and TB hospitals) Johannesburg, Durban, Transkei, Queenstown and the leprosy hospital in Lesotho. And what a person! Unlike the staff nurses, who tended to laugh at some Basotho customs, and the nurses aides, who were in some confusion caught between tradition and their acquaintance with western medicine, Sister Pauline took the tradition seriously and had a great insight into western minds. She was a prominent person in the community, and had her fingers in most pies and was always there when most needed, a veritable tower of strength.

STAFF NURSES.

There were between three and seven staff nurses, usually from the Lowlands. The Lowlanders generally were rather afraid of the mountains and thought that once at Mantšonyane they might never return. These nurses had courage, accepting the difficult conditions, but visits home were precious to them and needed at least five days.

The trained nurses did the normal maternity services, assisted in outpatients and theatre, undertook health education, immunisations, dispensing, difficult dressings, took charge of the inpatients and did some outreach work.

NURSE ASSISTANTS.

Many of the nurse assistants had been there for years. There were nine, mostly local people, whose education had stopped before high school. All but one spoke English. They looked after the inpatients, did simple dressings, washed the babies, assisted at deliveries, dispensed medicines, registered outpatients, tube fed the premature babies, and assisted at outstation clinics. A few went on to train as enrolled nurses.

The nurses were all very dedicated, and would do anything they could to help, they would stand in in an emergency, and were keen to learn, as I discovered when giving them lectures! Their understanding and presentation of the health care were of vital importance in the development of the hospital's medical service, as the community gradually gained confidence in it.

There were other things besides work. There were daily prayers in the chapel and on the ward. Sometimes there were feasts, or a game of basketball with the Waiting Mothers. (This game was rather popular when there were too many mothers-in-waiting for the limited accommodation!) One year we thought we might do a Nativity play. All the staff gathered for Father Manyane to explain what this was. They said they had never heard of such a thing, and were dubious-Was this not blasphemous? It became known in English as 'The Game'. All the staff and the Long-stay patients were in it. It was to be part of the Christmas Mass, performed near the stone staff houses down the airstrip. 'Me Puseletso was Mary as she had a small baby. A clear flag was put up outside one of the huts to show it was an Inn (usually the sign that beer was available). The Game had a life of its own, and evolved independently:- the scenes might happen in different orders; Joseph used to choose different places to go to sleep so Gabriel would have to look for him; and there were spontaneous additions, as once, when the birth was announced the entire cast responded traditionally by yodelling, dancing and singing their thanksgiving. The sheep came to a few rehearsals, but the donkey only appeared on the day, and there were two of them. (I was told this was in case the first one refused!) On the day the Roman Catholics from Auray Mission joined us, the cast wore their finest garments, brilliant cloths, beads and hide blankets. A large truck arrived in the middle of the play. The driver was drunk, and as he climbed down, he frightened the sheep, which took off just before their scene! The shepherds rushed after them, with the angels in hot pursuit! The sheep came to rest on a small hillock nearby, and the resulting gathering was spectacular!

I have very vivid memories of Lesotho. They are of beauty, of the mountain people and their dignity, of hardships beyond our conceiving, remoteness, treacherous roads and ponies.

The terrain had such a profound influence on life that it is worth taking an imagined, but characteristic visit. Imagine that you are in Maseru, and were due to fly up the day before yesterday, but the escarpment was closed by a thick blanket of clouds impenetrable by even the biggest of the Lesotho Airways' planes, the twin-engine Islander. You have been to the Flying Doctor office at the airport and have spoken on the radio to Eve D'Aeth at Mantšonanye (no telephone). She said that it looked like raining and they were trying to fly an outpatient with a very badly broken leg; the road was very rough and muddy at the moment. They will drive the patient down if there is no flying in the morning, and you can be taken on the return journey.

Meanwhile you amuse yourself by strolling around Maseru, looking at the Deputy Prime Minister's cows grazing on the verges; donkeys being loaded with sacks of grain at Maseru Roller Mills; smart Basotho girls still wearing miniskirts and block shoes, with numerous hair plaits arranged in complicated designs; the colourful blankets worn by so many; smart officials driving round in mud-splattered Land Rovers; the open market selling clay beads, fat cakes, cotton prints, roasted mealies, herbalist's wares, charms, potions, feathers, bark, snake-skin and other unidentifiable objects; the chaotic bus station with people sleeping on the mountain, people waiting for the mud to dry and the bus to leave; the dark stores, modern offices, banks and supermarkets. You stand in the newly-finished stone Anglican cathedral absorbing the bare and beautiful simplicity.

The patient arrives in the land-rover-ambulance the following day, mid-morning, after a six-hour trip (instead of the usual three to three-and-a-half hours). You help the driver with his hastily compiled shopping list, two concrete lintels, shock absorbers, growing mash, petrol, post, stamps, beer, intravenous infusion fluids, fresh meat and vegetables, TB, drugs. Typhoid vaccine and 'find out why the coal hasn't come.' At 2pm, you check on the radio. It is still raining and off you go with only four-and-a-half hours of daylight left.

About fifteen miles from Maseru the tarmac ends. Michael, the driver, stops, and you hand him bits of wire and pliers as he puts on the four tyre chains. You pass near the historic fortress, Thaba Bosiu, (Mountain of Night), and see scars of erosion. A woman flags you down, she is going to Mantšonyane but there has been no bus. She squeezes in with her baby, baggage and one chicken. You have not even reached the Escarpment yet and there is an "Engage Low Gear" sign. Slowly you creep, bump and occasionally slide up Bushman's Pass. After that comes Molimo Nthuse (God Help Me Pass) and then Blue Mountain, the highest, (8,900ft) and the last of the road signs. The panorama of the mountains is breathe taking; bare, rugged chaotic peaks, deeply grooved and hidden here and there by storm clouds. Just below the road is a huddle of stone huts. The woman recognises someone and suddenly shouts to her through the closed windows! She is called 'Malerato, (Mother of Love). Her child wakes up, stares at you for a moment, then settles back to sleep; the chicken lets out an uncertain squawk. As you edge down into the Likalaneng valley, you meet a truck stuck fast. It has gouged out deep ruts and a group of men are digging and collecting stones. There are enough helpers so we press on although it is all Michael can do not to slide into the ruts. To complicate matters a herd boy of about ten, wearing boots that look six sizes too large, is dreamily driving a herd of oxen, sheep and mohair goats right towards you. Around here are a number of small villages half hidden in the folds of the mountains. One village has an oblong stone building that Michael says is the Anglican school, church and clinic all in one room. It is on your way up Robber's Pass that darkness falls and you lose a chain. You have long since slithered into the ruts and have become used to the sensation of being in a boat. But now you are really stuck. There is a landrover behind you and another vehicle with only one light coming down the Pass. While it is pulling you out there is a lot of chatting and Michael is able to lend some tools to fix a broken windscreen wiper. After another three-quarters of an hour, you see some lights – Marakabei village, with a Store and a generator. The Senqenyane River Bridge is impressive even in the dark, and you can hear the roar of the swollen river. The last pass is one of the worst, very steep and slippery as it hugs the mountainside. A few smallish rocks have fallen on to the road, and you pass any number of unscheduled streams. Michael entertains you with anecdotes, while you glance below you at the right hand edge and nothing but blackness beyond.

Surprisingly you reach the top, Cheche's Nek, and you now drop down towards Mantšonyane. Half a mile off the main road a cluster of lights suddenly appears. You have arrived.

This is typical of journeys on the mountain road!

I was privileged to visit Ha Khomari in Lesobeng several times; a vivid source of memories. I had ridden very little before: the first time John Maseli kindly took me and we seemed to trot nearly all the way – it took four-and-a-half hours and that was easily my quickest journey there. (Usually we took about seven hours.) That first time there were 171 patients. They came for ante-natal examination, to collect TB drugs, for family planning, for treatments of coughs, colds, skin infections, toothache (extractions were done outside as it was too dark inside the hut), urinary tract infections, STD's, well anything. What would happen if they became ill just after the monthly visit? Would they face the journey to Mantšonyane, or wait until next month?

It was on visits to remote areas like this that we saw so vividly the inadequacy of the hospital-based curative medicine. Some health education was undertaken, and the people listened. In response to one plea they set about constructing a pit latrine near th Ha Khomari clinic. It was a splendid sit-down design (not the more usual squat version), but had no door and opened onto the bridal path, so our use of it was duly noted!

One of my most memorable visits to Ha Khomari was with Ntate Egbert. We had missed a couple of months because of bad weather, and felt we had to go even though the ground was covered in snow. Surprisingly Ntate Egbert had never been there before. We thought that there would be very few patients so no nurse assistants came. It was my birthday, which I marked by falling off the horse soon after leaving the hospital! No harm was done, and we had a stunningly beautiful ride over Thaba Moea. On arrival, Ntate Egbert became transformed. He was no longer the one who ran to open doors for me, and always agreed, 'Yes mother'. He sat down and discoursed with Morena Khomari, while I waited on them. It was a wonderful experience of great dignity. The next day we had far more patients than expected. Ntate Egbert was very helpful, but shy, so a female patient we knew well, a local teacher, was given a crash course in dispensing and helping with the work.

For myself, the time at Mantšonyane was one of richness, with a constant awareness of support. It is hard to understand why I have been so fortunate, in being given this experience. I came with an inadequate and wavering faith, and was showered with blessings, and some answers to prayer that have always been there for me in dark times since. While I was there, the community saw a deepening trust of Western curative medicine under Brian and Siân, and the beginning of a trend towards preventative care, as the inadequacy of the curative approach was experienced. When Richard and Eve D'Aeth arrived the people were ready to begin development of a more extensive preventive programme, and the nurses were to play a key role in this.

Chapter 7. HELP FROM SOUTH AFRICA.
Richard D' Aeth writes about St. James' from December 1974 to November 1977:

The first question one has to answer when saying that one worked at St. James' Hospital Mantšonyane, in the mountains of Lesotho is, 'How on earth did you get there?' A more searching question would be, 'Why did you go there?'

The simple answer is, 'It just happened.' For me, for our family, it was a wonderful happening. I think I can tell you how it happened. However I am still not too certain, 'Why.'

I was the Dean of the residence for the medical students of the University of Natal, Durban, South Africa. On Sunday mornings Fr. David Wells or one of his colleagues from the Society of the Sacred Mission (SSM) would come to the residence to hold Mass in the residence's library. Eve (my wife), the children, and I usually attended.

'When can you come for dinner?' Eve and I asked him after service one Sunday. His Sunday morning visits were always rushed. 'Tomorrow,' David replied. It was over dinner that we talked with, and came to know more about this tall, thin rather angular and gaunt Australian who smoked constantly, and had a keen but dry sense of humour. As he chatted with Eve and me over after-dinner coffee and liqueur, we learned of his involvement as accountant, priest, and board member, with a mission hospital in Lesotho, St James' Hospital at Mantšonyane, situated at the end of the Mountain Road. David told us that the current physician had fulfilled his contract and was about to return to Britain. He went on to tell us that it was extremely difficult to recruit doctors to the hospital. This came as no surprise, as we knew from our work at the medical school that it was always hard to recruit physicians to remote rural areas.

I had become somewhat dissatisfied with the prevailing philosophy of providing health services. The thinking of the day was very physician-oriented, and did not serve the rural majority well. Rural health services were bad in South Africa; they could only be worse in the tiny, impoverished country of Lesotho.

Eve and I began, slowly at first, like a trickle, and then like a swelling stream, with growing earnestness, to think about the possibility of working in Lesotho and solving Fr. David's and the Hospital's problem. I could use the opportunity to emphasise community health, and place more responsibility for patient care with nurses (who, as I was to soon learn, were already doing a great deal).

On his next visit to Durban, David was again our guest. This time we talked seriously about working at St. James' Hospital. David, ever careful, thoughtful and sensitive, advised caution. He suggested that before we made any decision, we should spend four to six weeks at Mantšonyane to see what the place was like and see how the family, and in particular the children, took to the idea. He was equally anxious that the hospital staff find us compatible. They had never before had a South African physician.

During the next long university holiday we acted on David's suggestion of going for a working holiday. We left Durban mid-1975 and drove to Maseru. From there, we drove east 80 miles to Mantšonyane. We arrived at the hospital about teatime where Ros, the matron, warmly welcomed us. She showed us our accommodation, a house now vacant, but when there was one, used by the maintenance manager. After we had settled in, Ros gave us tea, introduced us to the staff, and showed us round the hospital. Brian, the doctor, and his wife Siân were out doing a clinic at the village of Ha Khomari, a six-hour horse ride away.

Brian and Siân returned in a day or so. Then the next day, after introductions all round, we started work, and I began to get a glimpse of the work that was being done. The ability of the nurses was impressive. It was remarkable how much they did and how much responsibility and initiative they took, especially when the doctor was away and there was no one to refer to. The nurses saw and treated patients with great competence.

Eve and I learned a great deal about the people and their customs. Patients paid about 50 cents per hospital visit and about R3-50(about £1-75) per day for a hospital stay. At times they could not afford this fee but treatment was never refused. Often we would have a patient return to the hospital of his own volition to tell us that he had been able to sell a sheep, or that he had been working on the South African gold mines, and could now pay his debt of some two or more years old.

A combination of Ros, Brian and Siân, the staff of St. James, the people served, Lesotho and the hospital itself – all of these mixed together, won us. We moved to Mantšonyane about three months later, not the eighteen months we had originally contemplated.

Siân and Brian were a difficult team to follow. They were quiet, efficient and superbly competent. Most importantly they were loved and respected. I soon learned that it was one thing to work at Mantšonyane with Brian, it was quite another to work as the only doctor. Without Ros' help and support, I do not know how I would have coped. As one small example, it was Ros who taught me how to extract teeth. It was one thing to teach anatomy and know the details of the structure of a tooth, it was quite another to know how to remove it from a patient's mouth.

Talking of teeth brings back the memory of a dentist. For a while we actually did have a dentist. The Private Health Association of Lesotho (PHAL), somehow or other managed to get a dentist, Barry Simmone, from Texas. He visited all the PHAL centres. Barry was charming, outgoing, and energetic. Every few years he took off from his practice to work for about six months in developing areas. He came complete with a portable dental rig and equipment and, of course his lovely Texan accent. When he wasn't busy doing work, of a nature we were quite incapable of performing, he taught us to do better dental work with the equipment and skills we had. He also entertained us with pictures of the dental work he had done in other places. The pictures were most emphatically not for dinner time showing. The work he had undertaken in various places was impressive and moving. He showed us some of the problems he had to cope with and the work he had done in a leper colony in some country where quite clearly the term 'leper' meant more than someone with leprosy. We were extraordinarily lucky to have him, for his skill, humanity, and his personality.

A question I needed to answer for myself, as well as for the community at large was, what did I want to achieve? How could I contribute to the solid foundations built, and the growth achieved by my predecessors? How could I continue to carry the hospital forward? Could I?

Preventative work is usually a hard sell in any society. It is quiet, unassuming, and lacks drama. It is particularly difficult to promote when life itself consists of an unforgiving struggle for survival, and where financial poverty is omnipresent. However, that is where my interest lay. We began to try to move to a preventative and to a community health model. As you will see, I pushed too hard and too fast in this direction. I had to learn to wait for opportunities.

Friday was *bakhachane* day (antenatal day) and always extremely busy. The mothers were always given something to take away with them. There was method behind this. In a place where people had so little, the powdered milk or cooking oil acted as an incentive to entice them back for subsequent visits.

Preventative obstetrics and early detection of obstetrical problems was high on our agenda. We discussed ways of ensuring that the antenatal records were plainly and simply seen in the patients' *bukana* (clinical record book). This we did by developing a highly visible stamp where the clinical record of the prenatal visit was clearly and easily recorded. This made monitoring a mother through her prenatal period simpler. Making these bookkeeping changes was the easy part. Our difficulty was educating patients in labour. Try as we might, we were seldom able to dissuade the mother from pushing, and pushing hard, from the onset of the very first contraction. We tried to teach them that there was a time for pushing, and to wait and not to push, a time to conserve strength. However, from mother to daughter through generations they were taught that they had to push right from the start. Push they did to the point of exhaustion. If a midwife was at the mother's side, she stopped but so often, the moment the midwife left, the mother would again start pushing. One can only hope that we dissuaded even one or two mothers from passing this belief to their daughters.

There was great faith in 'the doctor', and in *'ente'*, (injection). Knowing the capabilities of the nurses and that so much could be diagnosed and treated by them, I wanted the people to feel more comfortable with the nurses. I also wanted the nurses to know that they were capable of dealing with most of the problems. Patients did not like this; they wanted to see the doctor. Eventually we reached a kind of compromise on that score. It was a difficult issue for a number of reasons. Patient resistance was a major factor, and of no less importance, the nurses had their own work and we did not have the money (or accommodation) to take on additional staff.

Faith in an injection, regardless of what was injected, exposed people to abuse. There were quacks, even nearby, who would inject tiny doses of penicillin, "just to help them" (in fact, to get a substantial income). This faith in an injection was seriously abused and it was distressing. There was little one could do about this except to try to convince people that, where indicated, oral medicine was just as good. I feel some progress was made. At least I hope so.

My efforts in both these two directions were pursued too soon after my arrival and with too much enthusiasm on my part. People didn't like it. I had not allowed enough time for people to know me and trust me. I tried to do things differently far too fast. Ros and Fr. David came to my rescue, gently but firmly slowing me up. I needed to get used to the ways of the people of the mountains; I had a lot to learn.

The hospital's obvious area of weakness at the time was the lack of a skilled maintenance manager. Of course, as everyone knows, because you are a doctor at a mission hospital, without any training, you are (or are supposed to be) by osmosis or by some supernatural power, an expert on diesel engines, water pumps, vehicles, and generators – plus everything else! Nevertheless in spite of this doctor's supposed expertise, the machinery was showing serious signs of neglect. Someone knowledgeable was urgently needed.

There were a number o British International Voluntary Services (IVS) volunteers in Maseru.Lois, co-ordinator of the IVS programme used to visit them from time to time. I wrote to her to ask her if she could recruit a maintenance manager for us.We wanted someone who was skilled and who could show people how things could be done. On her next visit to Maseru she came up to visit us and see our situation for herself.

On this particular visit, two young volunteers who had come from South Africa were trying to take the shackle pin out from the rear leaf spring of the Land Rover (they indicated they knew what to do). In layman's terms, this pin holds the spring to the body of the vehicle. As we were walking round the compound, Lois remarked, 'Let's go over and see how they are doing'. We sauntered over to see them at work. The jack was placed under the axle to raise the vehicle while they hammered out the pin out with a sledgehammer. The jack should have been under the chassis to support the vehicle once the pin was out. Had the vehicle been jacked up as it should have been, the pin would have come out with a few blows from an ordinary sized hammer. When we got to them, the pin was almost out. We stopped them just in time. It just needed a few more blows before the pin would have popped out. Had this happened, the whole vehicle, unsupported as it was, would have collapsed on top of them. They would have been killed, crushed to death. We got our maintenance manager, Mark McPoland!

Mark quickly fitted into the life of the hospital, mixed with, and was liked by everyone. He was a mechanic with a special interest in diesel engines and he kept the engines and machinery going beautifully. He used to say, 'Diesel engines talk to you.'

One of the staff nurses working in the Marakabei clinic commented one day that she had been talking to a group of women, and talking about the importance of hand washing (typhoid was endemic). One of the women had replied, 'Of course you have to wash your hands, you are a nurse. I'm not, so I don't have to wash my hands.'

This remark started us thinking and planning. We were not getting across the educational barrier. Even if there was no language barrier, the staff nurses' education was a barrier we had to bridge. We had to get into the people, not just to them.

Staff Nurse Matšeliso from the children's clinic agreed to train a Village Health Worker (VHW). The concept was that we would approach the chief and people of a village, preferably a distant one where access to the hospital was difficult and the benefit of a VHW therefore potentially greater. We would ask the village to select someone they trusted; we would then invite that person to come to the hospital for about six months to learn very basic medicine and hygiene. The VHW would also emphasise proper feeding and would encourage mothers to have their children immunised. Her emphasis would be on prevention. The care she would or could give would be very basic, home medicine: nothing more. However, being from the village, she could also talk to people about basic hygiene and cross that barrier we had just experienced. We went to a village and spoke to the chieftainess and people. The village selected a mature middle aged lady who came to us to train. She was superb and an extremely capable person. By chance, just as she had finished her training, the chieftainess of her village, came to see us as there was a problem with gastro-enteritis. 'Could we please come and help them, so many of the children had gastro-enteritis?'

This seemed the perfect time to introduce the lady as a VHW back into her own village, so we agreed. Accordingly, a party of us left for the village, led by the chieftainess. Mark came with us for the ride. Unfortunately, the horse Mark was riding was taught by its previous owner to make a bee-line to all the beer huts and stop outside, just by the doorway. (The beer huts were identified by a white flag flying outside the door.) Mark's horse had never been taught correct etiquette. So with Mark not in control, the animal would canter on ahead, overtaking the chiefainess to get to the next beer hut. You simply do not ride past a chief. You absolutely do not!

After being overtaken a few times, the Chieftainess called out to Mark, 'Mark, I ride here (pointing to herself out in front), *Ntate Ngaka* (me) rides there (just behind her), *'Ma ngaka* (my wife) rides there (just behind me), and you Mark, you will ride - there! (At the back, pointing vigorously.)' Mark's horse understood perfectly, and that is how we proceeded for the rest of the six-hour journey.

At the village, the VHW soon had the women talking about hygiene and chanting, 'A spoonful of sugar, half a spoon of salt in a bottle of boiled water.' We felt that the scheme had worked. Sadly, for educational reasons, we realised that we would soon have to leave and so we didn't train another VHW. That was a pity as it seemed such a successful scheme.

One of the saddest days of the hospital was the day Ros left. She had given wonderful service to the hospital, both as an outstanding professional and a simply lovely friend. Her parting left a big hole, a hole in our hearts and as matron, a hole that would be difficult to fill.

After a while we were wonderfully lucky to have Sr. Tessa from the Community of the Holy Name (CHN) in Leribe (a small town in the lowlands of Lesotho). Sr Tessa was remarkable, loved by all, efficient and really good company. If I've said that about others at St. James, it is that St. James' attracted those exceptional people. It was Sr. Tessa who was to carry on the work of the hospital after we left, until another doctor could be found. She took on a very heavy responsibility and workload. It was not easy. What a wonderful person.

The constant figure in the hospital's history was Fr. David Wells. He appears in all our stories. He was a figure of stability, of understanding, of wisdom and strength. He was with the hospital, when John Maund was bishop of Lesotho, and after when Bishop Desmond Tutu replaced Bishop John, after the latter's retirement. David was there when Bishop Desmond left. Whatever the changes, David was the dependable and unfailing helmsman, and above all, a friend.

There were so many wonderful and memorable experiences. I simply cannot finish without recounting one.

The Department of Justice had decided to open a magistrate's court in the local village of *Ha Toka*. The opening by the Minister was to be followed by a reception at the local hotel. As one of the local dignitaries, I was invited to attend the reception. By chance, there were no vehicles at the hospital; the only way of getting there was on horseback. The question was what to do with the horse while I was at the reception. This was solved by one of the staff, Ntate Egbert. Ntate Egbert agreed to come and look after the horse. Accordingly, the two of us set off, riding, I in my three-piece suit, dressed suitably to meet the Minister of Justice. The Minister was not there, however, the King's brother, the Prince was, and we started talking. After the Prince and I had been speaking for a while, I indicated that as I was on call, I really should be getting back to the Hospital. The Prince asked how I had come, so I told him, and added that my horse was outside being looked after by Ntate Egbert. Together we went to the door. The darkness was inky black, while the stars and the milky way shone in the heavens above, simply brilliant, like sparklets frozen in space.

The Prince called, *'Pere!'* (Horse!).

Out of the blackness of the night a voice replied 'Coming my lord!' From the dark into the candlelight from the doorway appeared Ntate Egbert with our horses. Together we mounted and then rode off out of the candle light into the night, and back to the hospital. It was so medieval.

The difficulty in writing about St. James' Hospital and Mantšonyane is that it is hard to know how to end, when to stop writing about the many events and incidents of the place. So very much happened there. I know that for many, and most certainly for me, it was a watershed experience that changed my life forever. We saw and did things that made it impossible to go back to where we were before.

To have followed so many exceptional people, is a privilege. To have known and been able to have worked among, and with so many capable and extraordinary and loving people is in itself a great honour.

CHAPTER 8. DIFFICULT TIMES.

Sadly, for two and a half years, from November 1977 until May 1980, there was no resident doctor at St. James' Hospital. This presented major difficulties for the remaining staff. However, communications between Mantšonyane and the lowlands became little easier due to improvement of the Mountain Road, connecting the hospital with Maseru. The hospital was visited regularly by the doctors of the Lesotho Flying Doctor Service. During this period a heavy burden fell on the nursing staff, especially the stalwart matrons who carried on with great trepidation, with amazing skills in carrying out many tasks, which a doctor would normally have carried out.

The situation was far from satisfactory, but great efforts were made to keep the hospital functioning and to try to obtain the services of a resident doctor. It would probably have been easier if it had been possible to offer a realistic salary for the post. It was sacrifice enough to expect a doctor to give up several years to serve in a strange culture in an isolated place and fall behind in career prospects, without being crippled financially, especially for married doctors with young families!

In 1978 Ken Wells, the secretary, left the hospital but trained Claurina Sixishe, Sister Pauline's daughter, as secretary/book-keeper, before he left. Sister Tessa of the Community of the Holy Name, who had often assisted at the hospital for three month periods since 1972, giving welcome relief to the matrons, was asked in October 1977 to respond to a crisis at the hospital, when Barbara Shield had to return home to nurse her sick parents. There was no Mosotho staff nurse who was willing to take on the post of acting matron and so Bishop Tutu, who had succeeded John Maund as second Bishop of Lesotho two years earlier, asked the Community of the Holy Name to allow Sister Tessa to act as Matron, with the promise of a doctor, soon to replace Dr. D'Aeth, who was about to leave. To the joy of the staff who knew and loved Sister Tessa well, she arrived to take up the duty as temporary matron.

Sister Tessa comments:

It wasn't easy without a doctor, although we had radio contact, which was a help. I read textbooks between clinics! It was fortunate that we had no midwifery complications. I had loved going out to the clinics at Ha Mafa and Lesobeng on previous visits, but after Dr. D'Aeth left, it was really a case of getting on with things and praying that nothing too disastrous would happen. The nurses were very supportive and I relied on Sister Pauline's experience of the hospital and the people and on the nurses who translated for me in the clinics and on the wards. I had by this time, because of my annual visits, got used to treating wounds of various kinds and stitching them up, although severe head wounds presented more of a problem. If I had any anxiety over a patient, I did what I could and then transferred them to the Queen Elizabeth Hospital in Maseru. Seeing patients in the clinics and trying to make the right

diagnosis, I thought, was always a bit precarious. On the whole things were not too bad and it was always so pleasing to have patients come back feeling better.

I loathed having to deal with teeth and of course some patients waited until the pain had got so bad and their gums inflamed and teeth rotten, but their relief when the offending tooth was dealt with and they were given Penicillin, was very satisfactory. Again some were beyond my dealing and had to go to Maseru.

Poorly babies and children were not always easy, especially when it seemed things had been left too late, and they were almost 'in extremis' by the time they were brought to the hospital.

One vivid moment I recollect, was when a boy of about 9 years was brought to the hospital in a very ill state suffering from pneumonia, malnutrition, scabies, and dehydration. I was trying to get an intravenous drip up for him his veins were so collapsed, it was proving very difficult, and then to my surprise and delight the flying doctor arrived and came to the rescue. Sadly, the boy died in spite of our efforts and I went over to the doctor's house where I was living with two of the Leribe sisters and had a good weep.

I hated tapping fluid from men's hydroceles and was so afraid of getting it wrong but 'Deo Gratia' managed not to.

One Sunday afternoon we received a message that a lorry carrying several people from Maseru had overturned on the Mountain Road; amazingly none had been severely or fatally injured, but it was a case of all hands on deck to get them back to the hospital, treated and admitted if necessary. The off- duty staff were so good in coming in to help.

In July Sister Pauline Ebuse Sixishe, who had served the hospital faithfully for 15 years, retired. She did not however deprive the people of Lesotho of her expertise and knowledge and continued running an out- station clinic.

Sister Tessa, CHN stayed on as temporary matron for ten months, until in August 1978 when she had to leave due to ill health and return to the UK. Her tremendous contribution over a period of half a dozen years will never be forgotten by the Basotho. Not only did she render much needed nursing care but her presence at the hospital together with the Basotho sisters showed wonderful loving care, which was widely appreciated both by staff and patients. Sister Tessa, who recently provided the above account of her service at Mantšonyane, is now a member of the contemplative community of the Sisters of the Love of God at Oxford and in 1999, with two other sisters went to work at St. Isaac's Retreat, New Zealand.

St. James' was fortunate to have an immediate replacement for Sister Tessa in Miss Pippa Gaye, who had been working in Botswana. At the same time, Michael Bartlett arrived to work as administrator for 16 months. Mr P. Agland commenced building the new Maternity Ward, but as time went by without a doctor the building was postponed.

Pippa Gaye recounts:

One day a lady with a broken ankle arrived on horseback and had to be helped into a wheelchair. After having her ankle X-rayed and plastered she was most indignant that we would not allow her to ride home immediately! Five out of the six male beds, we have, are occupied by TB patients plus all three beds in the isolation ward. The Bromsgrove Female Ward was often overflowing onto mattresses on the floor. We see as many as three fractures in one morning.

Matron Pippa Gaye had to leave to undergo major throat surgery and Staff Nurse E.Phororo was asked to act as matron for the time being. She was the first Mosotho to hold this position and managed to hold things together until the first permanent Mosotho Matron, Veronica Khadi, was appointed in February 1980 as a secondment from the Government of Lesotho.

In the interim period Sister Marjorie Eileen from Sister Tessa's Community of the Holy Name acted as Matron for a time. She had worked in hospitals of the Church Missionary Society in Sierra Leone and Nigeria and so was no stranger to African medicine.

She recalls a very busy weekend:

A bus carrying returning Basotho miners from the Republic of South Africa plunged down the mountainside on a hairpin bend a few miles from the hospital, when it was snowing. I was called at midnight to prepare theatres, beds and mattresses on the floor. Patients then began to arrive. Many people helped with cars for transport and our ambulance was busy. We rendered first aid whilst awaiting the arrival of a doctor from Maseru. I remember putting thirty-two stitches in a poor miner's leg without any anaesthetic - he never uttered a word and his leg healed perfectly.

In January 1980 the Private Health Association of Lesotho embarked on a plan to help the hospital and the Lesotho Government also got involved. They promised to provide a doctor as soon as possible. In the mean time doctors of the Scott Hospital, Morija and Paray Hospital, Thaba Tseka, began to visit St James' on alternate weekends, to see patients and advise staff. In March 1980, the Lesotho Government fulfilled their promise and arranged for Dr. Walter Tjon-A-Ten and his wife, Annemie to come to the hospital from Holland. After two and a half years without a doctor this was cause for great rejoicing.

Full credit to all the staff, who pulled together magnificently to carry on the work during a prolonged period without a resident doctor. Special gratitude is due especially to Sister Tessa, Pippa Gaye and E. Phororo for their valiant and successful efforts to rise to the temporary but valuable role as Nurse Practitioners.

Chapter 9: RESCUE FROM THE NETHERLANDS.

Dr. Walther Tjon- A- Ten was sent from the Netherlands by an organisation called 'Medicus Mundi' and seconded by the Lesotho Government to work at St. James' Hospital. He worked for six weeks at Scott Hospital, Morija, to adjust to African Medicine with the French Protestant doctors who had always been most helpful to new doctors. While at Morija he had gone up each weekend with one of the doctors, from Friday to Sunday, before taking up duty as Medical Superintendent on 15th May 1980. He found that there were too many staff and too few patients. The maternity Ward and Staff House were half finished. Water and electricity supply, were non-existent. There was no hot water and both Land Rovers were broken down! Faced with this situation Walter and Matron Veronica Khadi set to work enthusiastically. Some staff were retired but all who left went without ill feeling towards the hospital.

In June 1980 Walther was able to report:

More work is now done by less staff than before. Within two weeks of our arrival we managed ourselves to provide hot water in the hospital. We are so proud of that! The generator and water pumps are fixed and we have no electricity or water problems any more. O yes, we had to rewire the staff quarters, because just before I arrived there had been a fire in the Matron's house because of faulty wiring. It has cost some money, but it will be safe for staff as well as patients.

One Land Rover has been fixed very cheaply but this is only temporary, so we have ordered a Toyota Land Cruiser, which should arrive soon.

The most important thing is that our hospital is becoming a real hospital again. The number of outpatients has increased and the wards are nearly full. The whole staff is enthusiastic and everyone is working hard. One of our Nurse Aids is now at St. Joseph's Roman Catholic Hospital at Roma for training in taking X Rays and our domestic supervisor is at the Scott hospital, Morija, also for training.

Everybody is determined to make it a real hospital by the end of the year and at the same time to reduce expenditure. We are using the colder weather, when the patients are fewer, to reorganise the hospital, so we offer patients the best medical treatment possible when we get busier in the spring.

I thank all friends of the hospital for past support and hope they will keep supporting and praying for us in the future, because we really need their help.

Three months later Walter reported:

The hospital flooring is completed but we have not yet performed any major operations. In spite of the fact that our Autoclave and X-Ray machine are not working, we have no reasons to complain and still

manage. We are getting very busy in the outpatient department and see about 250 patients each week (a 94% increase from when we arrived!). The wards are now usually full and sometimes overflowing.

On 15th August 1980, three months after our arrival, my wife and I were welcomed by the people of the area with a big 'Mokete' (Feast) attended by Bishop Philip Mokoku, (third bishop of Lesotho), together with the Minister of Health, the Ward Chief (the King's brother) and about 2000 local Basotho and many others. There were Sesotho dances and songs. Very nice, but the next Monday we had to work again and had about 70 outpatients.

Every day except Sunday, I do hospital ward rounds from 8.30 to 10.00 am. After that there are usually some problems with the maintenance department, the kitchen or administration to solve. They may be minor problems, but sometimes, major domestic problems which take a lot of Veronica's and my time. After a coffee break we have about 20 minutes to discuss things with the senior staff.

On Mondays, Tuesdays and Thursdays we deal with minor procedures including tooth extractions, plastering fractures and minor operations. Wednesday is administration day for writing letters, signing cheques and checking stocks of medicine and equipment. On Friday I always visit clinics. At The Government Health Centre, Marabei, I see about 50 patients, but on the first Friday I go to the other Government Clinic at Likalaneng first and then to Marakabei. On that day I see about 120 patients in all and return to the hospital at 7 to 8pm where there are problems to sort out and a few minor operations. I finish very late on that day.

At the end of September we are closing the Ha Khomari clinic at Lesobeng, as it requires 3 days away from the hospital to visit on horseback. Also the Government have opened a new clinic on the other side of the river and there is a doubly qualified staff nurse with regular visits by the flying doctors. However, between Lesobeng and the hospital we will re-open the clinic at Ha Mafa, only a few hours ride away. This clinic will be visited on the second Saturday of every month, returning on Sunday. Some of the Lesobeng patients will be able to attend this clinic which is about 4 hours ride for them.

We have restarted the Primary Health Care Programme with 'Pitsos' (meetings) with the people of many different villages to explain what the programme means. We have also invited the chiefs, teachers, civil servants and traditional doctors and many others from the villages to talk about the PHC Progamme on the 1st of October 1980.

In January 1981, Mr. Baba Sixishe (Sister Pauline's youngest son), who had served as local Maintenance Officer, left us and no replacement could be found.

In March 1981 Walther reported:

My wife is running the laboratory and helping out wherever needed with the administration and in the kitchen. She is also training one of the Nurse Aids, in laboratory work.

There is a now a co-ordinator for the Village Health Workers who are to become responsible for the PHC Programme in the Mantšonyane Health Service Area, (HSA)

We have built a pigsty and a new stable is being built.

A generous donation from the Netherlands has enabled us to purchase a new autoclave.

Walther and Annemie produced their first baby in June 1981. Annemie started to teach the PHC team to make hand puppets and to perform a puppet show to illustrate good health to mothers at the Under-Fives clinic. Annemie also taught the Nurse Aids English on four evenings a week.

In August 1981 the staff house was completed together with the coal shed, which prevented the odd bag of coal going missing. The ablution block for maternity patients was also finished

Walther recounts:

Very important and indispensable people around the hospital are five maintenance men. They have to cope with burst pipes in the winter, which produce a beautiful fountain in the middle of the compound; an area where we do not need water! The men have to run up and down to the well to stop the pump and then up to the tank to stop the flow of water through the pipes. Only then can they start repairing the leak, which sometimes, with all the digging involved, takes them a whole day.

The maintenance men are also responsible for everything which is broken or damaged - a generator, a car or a cupboard. They also take care of the garden where cabbage, kale, sprouts and carrots are grown and supply the hospital well into the winter. The same team also take care of our animals: chickens, goats sheep and horses and hopefully, very soon some pigs. Veronica Khadi stayed on as matron until the end of 1981 and trained Mrs Puthi Banda to take her place.

In January 1982, Mr Willem van der Werff arrived from the Netherlands to supervise the maintenance work.

In February 1982 a second Village Health Worker's course took place with 19 people from seven villages being trained.

In July 1982 Under-Fives clinics were at Ha Mafa and Likalaneng.

Mrs Janet Rakhetla took over as matron from Mrs Puthi Banda who had served seven months.

In November Walther talked about some of the patients treated:

A girl called Pontšo, aged 16, was admitted to hospital. She walked around throwing things and making a thorough nuisance of herself. After four days we wanted to send her to the mental hospital in Maseru, but her parents objected and took her away to a traditional doctor and nothing further was heard about her.

[This was a possible case of possession by an evil spirit, which we had occasionally seen in the 1960's and treated successfully by the Laying of Hands with Prayer in the Name of Jesus - Editor.]

Walther continues

At Marakabei Clinic I examined a severely dehydrated child of three months of age with malnutrition. The little soul weighed only four pounds. We took her back to St. James' and, with some difficulty, put in an intravenous drip to re-hydrate her and then commenced feeding her on powdered milk as her mother had no milk of her own. After 6 weeks she weighed eight pounds, gaining weight every day until ready to go home.

To us it seems far -fetched for people to talk about 'Health for All' by the year 2000! Whether we will reach this goal in our area, I do not know, but through the work of our PHC we are doing our very best.

In April 1983 Walther reported:

Our new Maternity Ward was completed last year, in spite of many difficulties, what a relief! It is a beautiful brown building with yellow windows and door frames and a dark red roof. It looks very fine. It is light and quite warm in the winter. Bishop Philip Mokuku will officially open the ward but we hope to admit our first 'Batsoetse' (newly delivered mothers) almost immediately.

Willem van der Werff has been enthusiastically busy in our garden, so that everybody has decided to copy him. I have never seen so many garden plots in the hospital grounds, something I would never have imagined a year ago.

Our PHC Programme is functioning well although progress is slow; it is strange to many people, the importance of clean drinking water or a latrine. Sometimes things go seriously wrong as recently at Ha Mahlong nearby. A polluted well caused a Typhoid fever outbreak with 21 sufferers being admitted to hospital. Some of them died with a perforated bowel. Many others in the village were taken ill, but in spite of all the efforts of our PHC staff and Village Health Workers they refused to come to hospital. Some of them died at home. A father brought his two children to be treated. We asked where the mother was as one of the children was quite small. She was at home and a week later we heard she had died. When the children were cured they were collected by the father, but he himself returned three weeks later complaining of severe abdominal pains, having been unwell for two weeks. We admitted him for treatment, but he died two days later.

Such sad incidents make us feel that we would like to buy the materials and make the well safe ourselves. But experience has shown us that this is not the right way to go about things. It has proved much better to let the people collect the money for the materials themselves and this they will only do, when they realise the importance of the project.

We, of course, will help all we can when they come to this point. We offer information and practical help when the materials are on-site. The whole process takes a long time and sometimes it takes only a disaster, as I have described, to motivate the people into doing something. Without this motivation we have found that no protected well is properly maintained or what is even worse, people actually break down what has been built! In July our matron, Janet Rakhetla left and it has proved difficult to replace her.

In October 1983 Annemie Tjohn-A-Ten wrote to supporters:

We find that after three and a half years, we are grateful for all the difficult times we have had because it has taught us a lot about ourselves and it has strengthened our relationship. We recall disasters but we can see them in proportion as we have been able to overcome them with your help, although at the time one sometimes felt it was too much to handle.

Our latest disaster was on the 22nd September 1983 when St. James' Hospital, St. James' Mission and the villages of Ha Chooko and Ha Toka were hit by a tornado (setsokotsane). The damages the hospital suffered were: a collapsed store room, the laundry roof blown off which hit the new maternity block, making a hole, the outside corridor of the nurses' home blew away, the roof of the chapel trembled loose, the roof of the staff nurses' rondavel was lifted, the roof of the PHC nurses' house was partially blown off, the roof of the domestics' quarters damaged, the ceiling of the kitchen trembled loose, as did the roof of matron's cottage and the stable collapsed.

It was quite a frightening experience, but we were fortunate to have immediate help from the community architect and his builders, who were working on the new doctor's house, to do the most urgent repairs. The hospital looked black with dust and sand. Everybody worked hard to clean up the mess and the big repairing from insurance will soon be completed. After three and a half years with St. James' Hospital it will not be easy to say goodbye. We have in a way 'grown up' here. Our daughter, Paivi, now almost two and a half years, is speaking Sesotho even better than Dutch, our language!

Let Walther have the last word:

From all of us here at the hospital we would like to thank you all for your help, for your prayers and your donations. May God bless you all for all your kindness! Many of the past problems such as finding qualified staff and money to run the hospital have remained unchanged, but we are confident that you will continue to help as you have done in the past.

Walther and Annemie completed four years work in March 1984. St. James' Hospital will always owe a great debt of gratitude to them for rejuvenating its work so wonderfully and also for firmly establishing the Primary Health Care Programme.

CHAPTER 10. SUSTAINED HELP FROM THE NETHERLANDS.

Continuity of care from the Netherlands was ensured when Dr. Jan A. Vorisek and his wife arrived at Mantšonyane in October 1983 Jan became the seventh Medical Superintendent of St. James' Hospital in January 1984. It was a smooth hand-over with Walther still around until March. So often in the past there had not been such a useful overlap of doctors which in this case proved a marvellous opportunity for helping the new doctor with all sorts of practical advise of great benefit.

The hospital chapel of 'the Divine Compassion and St. Barnabas', which had been the focus of worship and inspiration was, after much consideration, converted and modified into a residence for a second doctor, who was to head the development of the Primary Health Programme as an important aspect of the work. For the first 9 months or so Jan Vorisek would still be the sole doctor and combine the jobs of Medical Superintendent and Director of the PHC Programme.

It seemed strange to supporters that the Chapel should be put to such a different use; but the terrible hurricane of 1983 had totally decimated St. James' Church and Mission across the river at Ha Chooko. There were plans ahead to rebuild the Church, Mission and School alongside the hospital, thus centralising activities on the same side of the river near the end of the Mountain Road. There would therefore be a large new church near the hospital and a new small chapel was to be attached to the rear of the hospital. In fact the beautiful stone altar of the old chapel was rebuilt in the new chapel, the sanctuary lamp now hangs in the new St. James' Church and the huge wooden cross is in the vestry of the new church.

Dr. Jan Vorisek (the surname will continued to be used to avoid confusion with Dr. Jan Voskens who came later) describes his new residence, the converted chapel:

It was painted bright yellow and orange while the new chapel attached to the hospital is red and pink in the shape of a rondavel. I think the Flying Doctor Service can find us now, even in the fog!

Looking around, we have a well run hospital with a competent staff headed by Matron Veronica M. Khadi, who has happily returned to work here and is well known for her utmost confidence and fervour.

Dr. Tjohn-A-Ten certainly did a tremendous piece of work here, but created some new problems in that with the hospital improved and the PHC Programme in full operation, it had become difficult to supervise and co-ordinate both, in addition to administrative duties, which take a lot of time, involving meetings in Maseru and Thaba Tseka. Fortunately there is hope of the arrival of a second doctor soon.

In April 1984 our hospital again experienced a Typhoid Fever outbreak. Last year the main sources of infection were Ha Mahlong and Ha Mafa, both with unprotected springs. This year we managed to

persuade the people of Ha Mahlong, which is quite near to us, to protect their water supply from contamination, but despite strenuous efforts the people of Ha Mafa remained stubborn. So up to now 20 new typhoid cases have been admitted from Ha Mafa alone, but none from Ha Mahlong!

In April also we held a workshop for 18 chiefs of the area to prevent misunderstanding about health problems and possible solutions. This is a slow process and we must not be discouraged, so that with all efforts and the help of God, we will ultimately succeed in the long run.

In August 1984 Dr. Jan Voskens and his wife, E. Bernink, finally arrived from the Netherlands. As a second doctor he was very welcome. Dr. Voskens (another Jan) is to be in charge of the PHC Programme. This will enable me to give less divided attention to the running of the hospital. With Dr. Voskens help we hope to extend the health services closer to the people and also to expand preventive health activities at all levels. More mobile (later called semi-permanent) clinics and school visits will be possible. Immunisations will be brought more to the villages instead of the people from far places coming (or not coming) to us for vaccinations.

Dr. Voskens' wife is an experienced physiotherapist and is keen to visit other hospitals on a monthly basis to lecture the nurses on simple physiotherapy. Scott Hospital, Morija, St Joseph's Hospital, Roma and the Maloti Hospital, Mapoteng together with Paray Hospital, Thaba Tseka, have all expressed interest in the scheme, which will be co-ordinated by the Private Hospital's Association of Lesotho (PHAL) to which all mission hospitals belong. We also report that the hospital roof was repaired and the insulation of the walls improved. Hospital and staff houses are now provided with very efficient solar heating to save on fuel consumption.

Another major undertaking is the renovation of the Training Centre (the original prefabricated staff house of the 1961 was in poor shape after 23 years). By redesigning the building we created space for 26 beds, a large lecture room, kitchen, toilets and washing facilities, by exchanging the prefabricated walls and replacing worn out pieces. The whole renovation has been done under the supervision of Mr. Willem van der Werff and his friend Kee-Jan Delst. We now look forward to the first Village Health Workers course soon to take place in the renovated Training Centre. During the renovation we continued to organise courses for the VHWs, Traditional Birth Attendants, (TBAs), teachers and chiefs.

A real major undertaking will be to build a new Marakabei Health Centre, taken over from the Government of Lesotho. The old building, erected 30 years ago, of corrugated iron, is literally falling to pieces. Had we not had such devoted staff there, braving heavy rains and cold winters, the clinic would have been closed long ago. A proper stone building and staff quarters will be built with the help of our friends.

Sadly, last month we lost three of our four horses within a short time. Two died of horse sickness and one broke its back. We are desperately trying to replace these as most of the PHC activities depend on this mode of transport.

In November 1984 Dr. Sam Moore from Scott Hospital held his first eye clinic at St. James' and saw 86 patients and performed six cataract operations.

In July 1985 Dr. Jan Vorisek reported further:

The year 1985 had a bad start after a severe night frost destroyed most of the mountain crops. In addition we were hit by a series of road accidents in which some of our friends lost their lives.

Our own hospital Four Wheel Drive vehicle, returning from a clinic visit, rolled over down the mountain due to collapse of the road caused by heavy rain. Fortunately no one was badly injured due to low speed, but the vehicle was extensively damaged. It took six weeks to recover the vehicle and another six weeks to transport it and have it repaired.

Another problem was the breakdown of our water supply system. Both engines successively gave up, only to be replaced by the wrong one. The old water pump then refused to produce more than a trickle of water and when replaced by a standby new pump, the pipes decided to burst, not having been used to such a show of power. Anyhow, we now have water again! However, we also have electric light and both generators are working. These problems could have been more easily solved if we had a skilled maintenance man. Unfortunately Mr. Vander Werff left in December 1984 and we have not yet been able to replace him.

Despite all these difficulties the hospital is moving ahead. Patient attendances are ever increasing and services are expanding. New laporoscopic equipment is now in use and we are able to carry out blood grouping.

Dr. and Mrs. Voskens have settled very well. Mrs. Voskens has commenced physiotherapy instruction in three other hospitals as well as our own. This is a good contact to have. Also, I recently visited parishes in the Diocese of Johannesburg, South Africa, which has a close link with Lesotho.

Another contact has been with the Roman Catholic Mission at Ha Nyane, better known as Auray Mission. We now have a strong co-operation with their dispensary and mission due to the keen interest by Father Bane, the priest in charge. Under-Fives and Ante-natal clinics have been started there with good response without a drop in attendance at the hospital, which is less than an hour's ride away.

Our problem with horses is solved. We now have three strong ones and two of them pregnant! The third horse is a powerful stallion, as one of our staff recently experienced, with a few broken ribs, although a skilled horseman.

In October 1985 a four-year Government water project was begun which is based at the hospital. A dam is to be built across the Mantšonyane River generating electricity to boost the national grid. This will provide a useful cheaper supply to the hospital.

In January 1986 Jan Voskens describes some of the difficulties and problems:

In the middle of the night a knock on the window wakes up the doctor on duty. The night-watchman gives him the message that he is needed in the hospital. A young mother has come with her premature twins born three days ago in the village at Lesobeng, three hour's ride away - they were born two months too early and their weight less than three pounds. The long journey has made them dehydrated in the heat and so despite all our efforts the smallest twin died within a few hours. The other one, tube fed and kept warm between the breasts of the mother is struggling for its life. We have no incubator yet and no intensive care possibilities, only limited means and dedicated nurses. We know his chances are small but we keep on trying our best.

In June 1986 Jan Vorisek wrote:

It seems this year will be 'A Year of Training Courses' for Village Health Workers, Traditional Healers as well as courses specially designed to combat childhood communicable diseases and the need for Family Planning. There will be 18 courses in all! As our staff and transport resources are limited, some courses will take place at the clinics - not an easy task. A course is planned for teachers at Ha Lephoi clinic in Lesobeng next week. Our FWD vehicle had to make two trips there to transport all the necessary items of mattresses, blankets, food and coal etc. On the second trip it got stuck in the snow and it took the occupants hours to get mobile. If it starts snowing again we may have to cancel the courses altogether.

As the hospital was recently connected to the electricity mains, some services were improved and we hope running costs will be lower.

On 26th May, many of the hospital staff went to Maseru to join in the celebrations commemorating the 25th anniversary of Bishop Philip's ordination to the priesthood by Bishop Maund in the year that the hospital project first started. Twenty- four of our staff attended the Mass and the joyful celebrations afterwards. For some of the staff it was their first visit in their lives to Maseru. They were fascinated by the traffic lights and the confusion caused by them, the size of the buildings and the street life. As our three car loads returned to Mantšonyane, it meant back to normal life again, to the future, the future of our staff and hopefully to the Mantšonyane area.

From August to October 1986 Dr. Jan Vorisek and his family went on home leave during which he visited many donors of the hospital. On their return they were accompanied by a new young Vorisek, Thomas, who was born in the Netherlands just before their return to Lesotho.

During the Vorisek's furlough Jan Voskens had to combine his care of the PHC with the duties of Medical Superintendent.

He reported, as follows:

Three of our staff nurses had left in 1985 and 'Me Moeno, our oldest nurse in age left us early in 1986. We struggle to keep up with government salaries, which are more attractive to new nurses.

Late in 1986 we were pleased to include, at last, a Premature Baby Unit in an enlarged nursery together with an incubator - powered by mains electricity, but with a battery backup. We also now have a Waiting Mother's Lodge, next to the Maternity Ward.

In January 1987 Dr. Jan Voskens reported:

Our new maintenance Officer, Mr. Oliver Conway, arrived with his wife. He will share his time between us and Semonkong Hospital. Ntate Phetiso will be trained to take over this work.

In March 1987, the new 14 bedded male ward (the converted old laundry) and the new laundry were officially opened by Dr. S. T. Makenete and blessed by Assistant Bishop Donald Nestor. The old male ward was now to be used for isolation purposes.

In August 1987 Dr. Voskens reported further:

The winter this year was one of the coldest on record with temperatures going down to 18 degrees Celsius below freezing. A hard wind kept blowing from the south one night, causing serious damage to water pipes and pump. The water pipe in the roof burst in six places and the wards were flooded, when the ceiling came down. At the same time two non-return valves made out of massive steel alloy, broke into pieces due to expansion of the ice. Last month snow covered the mountains and the hospital with a splendid white mantle. For a few days the hospital and the area were inaccessible because of the snow and ice.

In October 1987 St. James' said a sad goodbye to Dr. Jan Vorisek who completed his contract after four years devoted service as seventh Medical Superintendent of the hospital. At his farewell party he was honoured by the presence of Bishop Philip and Bishop Donald, many chiefs and local people. An ox, meant to be the main dish of the feast, took to its heels and vanished one night, anticipating his fate. After a long search he was found some 12 miles away. So the feast was a success and the staff were able to show their thankfulness for Jan Vorisek's work of improving the hospital so remarkably.

During 1987 the Staff Nurses rondavels were renovated and extended with solar heating for hot water.

Matron Veronica Khadi comments:

The end of 1987 was very busy. The work carried out during the last quarter doubled. We are proud of our nurses for the good work they did to help Dr. Voskens, the only doctor left. He had to care for the hospital as well as the monthly visits to seven clinics. The nurses screened all the outpatients and the first ante- natal visits, usually seen by the doctor. We were glad of the services of Mr. Klass Jan Kamminga, a medical student who helped us a lot. He came from the Netherlands, as did Dr. Marcel Annceaux, who arrived on the 26th December as a temporary relief for Dr. Voskens, who had been on his own for three months and always on duty unless away at a clinic or meetings.

Unfortunately Dr. Voskens was unable to take a break because he suddenly felt ill and had to go to bed. He continued to help solve medical and administrative problems but was not getting the rest he needed in spite of good nursing care. It was decided that he should go to Masite Priory in the Lowlands where the sisters of the Precious Blood could care for him.

In his absence Fr. David Wells did all the financial administration at the end of the year. It had already been arranged for Dr. Marcel to go to the QE II Hospital in Maseru for familiarisation with the local medical scene. This left the medical student, Klaas to prepare and present patients for the doctor from Paray Hospital, who came over from Thaba Tseka.

.Dr. Jan Voskens recovered and returned to St. James'. In his last newsletter he expressed a mixture of sentiments as follows:

We have enjoyed every moment of working for four years at Mantšonyane! At times we struggled in hardship and how good it is to see the hospital growing and flourishing; the increasing number of patients, the opening of new wards, the expanding network of clinics and other primary health care activities. In fact St. James' has developed into a full-sized health facility after a difficult 25 years, as we approach the anniversary of the official opening on 7th September, 1988. Though we are looking forward to this great event, we are extremely concerned about the future survival of our hospital. In fact we are in the midst of a very critical and serious financial crisis. We have been forced to increase our staff salaries, to keep in line with the lately revised Government salaries. This means an increase of 60% of our present salary budget. If we don't do this we will lose staff and so the hospital board has decided to draw on our resources - even so this will only see us through six months.

Together with other Mission Hospitals and all the Heads of Churches we have taken the ultimate step of addressing the King and calling for immediate financial support from the Government. There is a real possibility that our hospital and others will have to close if nothing happens. We feel defeated and only ask for a miracle!

I appeal to all our friends to prevent closure of St. James' Hospital. We need 100 000 Maloti (£25 000) to cover the deficit for this year alone.

Jan Voskens had been most active in extending the PHC Programme and his wife, Els, had trained assistants to do laboratory work and physiotherapy. They left an indelible mark on the hospital's history, which at this point was threatened with extinction.

Dr. Paul Borgdorff had arrived in April 1988 and took over as Medical Superintendent in July 1988, when Dr. Jan Voskens left. In his first letter he reported triumphantly:

We have experienced that miracles do happen! Financial support has come from all over the world, north and south. Generous support came from the USPG and other organisations as well as many individuals. In their efforts to keep St. James' Hospital going. Indeed we can breathe again, for this year we do not have to use any money from our meagre reserves and we can even cover the expenditure for part of next year.

The greatest event this year was of course the celebration of the 25th anniversary held on the 2nd of September 1988 (five days before the actual day of the opening in 1963). We were honoured by the visit of His Grace, Archbishop Desmond Tutu of the Church of the Province of Southern Africa (Second Bishop of Lesotho).

His Highness, King Moshoeshoe II of Lesotho was also present as was the long serving friend of the hospital, Dr, S. T. Makenete, Minister of Health, as well as representatives of the Council of Ministers of the Lesotho Government.

Mass was celebrated in the morning by His Grace and in the afternoon many officials spoke encouraging words to the staff and the 600 people gathered for the celebration.

We hope we will be given many years to go on with the work that is allocated to us.

In October 1988 we held a three day meeting with representatives from all over the district (Chiefs, teachers, agricultural experts, Village Health Workers, clinic nurses and hospital staff) to set priorities for the development of health related facilities during the next 5 years. It was a very inspiring meeting. We realised that health is regarded as very important by the people in our Health Service Area. We saw that they appreciate the way we are trying to promote health by curative and preventive services. Lack of good roads was definitely problem number one, but also the shortage of clinics and health personnel ranked high on the list of priorities. We found the meeting very motivating in formulating a 'Five Year Plan', for continuing and expanding our work. Our report was sent to 'The Health Population and Nutrition Project', financed by the World Bank.

In January 1989 Mr. Oliver Conway, our maintenance Officer, completed his two years valuable service but no replacement has yet been found.

In February 1989, we welcomed back Klaas Jan Kamminga, now a qualified doctor together with his wife, Jos, to serve again with us for twelve months.

In April 1989, the rewiring of the hospital was completed. A new three phase system has replaced the old single phase one. It was carried out by a voluntary electrician through 'Stichting Netherland–Lesotho'. Now the whole hospital compound has electricity 24 hours a day and each house has a meter. Also in April, our X-ray machine broke down and the tube had to be sent to Johannesburg for replacement(R 7 000-£1 750).

I have some good news. We have started the protection of two big springs for the hospital water supply. This will be expensive as both springs require a lot of piping to reach the storage tanks. Thanks are due to the Lesotho-Durham Link and the European Community for financing this essential project.

At present our shortage of nurses is critical- we have only one who can do midwifery. We hope that it will be easier to attract nurses with the salaries we are now paying, which are on a level with the Government ones, although the Government are only paying 80% of this.

In January 1990 Paul Borgdorff reports further progress:

In January we said goodbye to Dr. Klaas Kamminga who had worked on the PHC Programme for a year and Jos who had worked in the physiotherapy department of the hospital.

In February 1990 our new Administration Block, which had taken five months to build, was opened by the Minister of Health and blessed by Bishop Donald, vice- chairman of the hospital board in the presence of the donors: the EEC, Lesotho-Durham Link, the German Ambassador and the British High Commissioner. This extension gives us opportunity to improve the Outpatient Department with a second consulting room and a larger dressing room, where two patients can be treated at the same time. We are grateful to the Lion's Club Frankfurt for this improvement.

On the same day, the two new springs were officially opened due to the generosity of the Lesotho-Durham Link and the British High Commissioner. The kitchen was re-tiled and a new ceiling put in at the same time. Mr. Mielin, a retired builder from the Netherlands, sponsored by the Netherlands Management Consultancy Programme of The Hague, arrived. He was to supervise the building of the new staff quarters, with twelve units. He was also to train our maintenance staff.

In April 1990, 'Dienst over Grenzen' (DOG) arranged for another Dutch doctor, Paul H. Breedveld and his wife to come to St. James' on a three year contract. Dr. Breedveld took over the duty as director of the PHC Programme and José, a nutritionist, upgraded the activity of the hospital kitchen and stock taking in the hospital and clinics as well as carrying out nutritional education.

During July and August Dr. Paul Bordorff went on home leave and also visited the UK and Germany, discussing the hospital with supporters, leaving Dr. Paul Breedveld in sole charge of the hospital and PHC.

The hospital board agreed to increase patient fees to supplement income but still far short of the actual cost of care and drugs.

In 1990 the operating theatre was renovated to full hygienic standards. A further course for Traditional Healers was held at Auray Mission; it was mainly spiritual in coverage and was much appreciated by those who attended. In the same year both outpatients and deliveries increased, in spite of fee increases.

In 1991 the greatest concern was again financial. In spite of 50% Government grants towards nurses' salaries, PHAL including our bishop and other church leaders requested the government to take over payment of all mission hospital staff. This was granted in April 1991 but sustained for only twelve months. However this prevented the imminent closure of many mission hospitals.

Paul Borgdorff reported in January 1991:

Mr. Mielin left us after completing the new block of houses with running water and electricity, for the junior staff.

After many years of seeking financial support for a refrigerated mortuary, the money has come from the Canadian Embassy. This means, that families whose men work in the mines can postpone the funeral.

The recruiting of nursing staff is still difficult and we continue to rely on Nurse Assistants who have only one year's formal training. High school leavers are employed in the laboratory and drugs store. This helps to alleviate the heavy workload of nurses and doctors.

The skill of nurses practising physiotherapy has continued to improve and they have benefited from attending two nation-wide workshops.

Pregnant women are still encouraged to attend hospital for delivery as TBAs supervise so few deliveries. We do however give TBAs training and help them to recognise problems.

Modern Family Planning is not widely accepted and rumours about side effects persist. Husbands are a main target group as they are often unaware of the benefits of limiting family size or that children can be well spaced.

Health Education sessions are held when we visit schools, attend community meetings, run training courses for VHWs and on our rounds to mothers and TB patients. This enables us to reach as many people in the community as possible. We cover information about immunisation, weaning, food, alcoholism, smoking, family planning, AIDS and breast - feeding.

We have been delighted at the good attendance of VHWs at refresher courses but attendance by Traditional Healers has been poor – unfortunately they fear that we will check them for their government

licences, but this is not the case. Those who do attend, often enter into general and open discussion, which is appreciated by all

On the 28th of February 1991 Nursing Officer 'Mathato Phororo completed more than fifteen years committed service to the hospital.

In July 1991 Senior Nursing Officer, Lebajoa, completed an 18 month diploma course in nursing administration and community service at the University of Western Cape. Nursing Sister Lepheana passed a one-year course for Nurse Clinicians at the National Training Centre and took charge of the clinic at Ha Lephoi.

In October 1991 Dr. Paul Borgdorff, Medical Superintendent, married a Mosotho, 'Mamolepa Lebotsa.

In January 1992 Nursing Sister P. Matete went for a year's training in Public Health, sponsored by the World Council of Churches.

In February 1992 baby Eva Puleng (Born in the rain) was born to Dr. Paul and José Breedveld.

In March 1992 a new Ultra-Sound Machine was donated by the Lion's Club, Frankfurt and enabled 455 scans for antenatal diagnosis to be performed, before the end of the year.

In April 1992 Dr. and Mrs Paul Borgdorff returned to the Netherlands, completing over four years most valued service to the hospital. Paul was to study Gynaecology.

In June a new machine for Nitrous Oxide anaesthesia and artificial respiration was donated by the Schumacher-Kramer Foundation of the Netherlands.

From August to October Dr. Paul Breedveld and José went on furlough and Dr. Geoff Protheroe visited St. James' for a few days each week from Tebellong Hospital.

From August to December 1992 Dr. Raol Hamers was sent from the Netherlands, through the DOG to act as a relief doctor.

Dr. Barbara Holoubek from Germany, was sponsored by her parents to serve from November 1992 to April 1993.

At this time the large PHC hall was used for a weekly service on Wednesday morning. At the end of January 1993 Dr. E. Oosterhuis arrived to be new Medical Superintendent with his wife.

In April 1993 the Breedvelds left the hospital after three years much appreciated service. The staff gave them a farewell party when they were thanked for all that they had done for the hospital and especially for the surrounding community. As it was autumn they left wearing traditional Basotho blankets and hats.

In his last letter, Dr. Paul Breedveld wrote:

We leave Lesotho with mixed feelings since we have enjoyed our stay very much and will treasure the good memories we have of serving the hospital.

In June 1993 Dr. Liesbeth Meuwissen and her husband, Erik van de Giesson, a water engineer, joined the staff. Liesbeth was the first lady doctor to serve for a long period and became director of the PHC Programme and Erik became Project Co-ordinator for the Lesobeng Spring Protection project, involving 27 villages.

In July Dr. Oosterhuis reported that they were busy in the hospital with patients sleeping on mattresses on the floor. With all the extra washing, they were pleased to have a new washing machine, donated by the Lion's Club, Frankfurt, Germany. Washing 35 pounds of clothes and linen was just a matter of pushing a button, waiting an hour and then hanging them out in the sun.

At this time a new and better stove was installed in the hospital and the Netherlands Embassy financed the fencing of the airstrip, which made it much safer for landing.

In October Mr. B. Motjeane, the laboratory assistant went to Maseru for training in the detection of Acid- fast bacilli in sputum smears which would greatly improve the diagnosis of TB.

Two new Van Hamel's incubators, which were easy to operate, were installed. The smallest baby to survive weighed two pounds at birth and left the hospital weighing five pounds!

At Christmas 1993 the staff did a round of the wards, each holding a lighted candle, while the Gospel of the birth of Christ was brought to the patients in readings, preaching and communal singing. Small parcels were handed out to the patients as a result of the kindness of the staff of the Standard Bank, Maseru.

The bed occupancy rose in 1993 to 798, the highest yet. The year also closed with a small profit, not allowing for depreciation of vehicles. Mrs Oosterhuis ran a knitting and sewing class for staff and waiting mothers, which was well attended.

However, all was not well at St. James' Hospital in 1994. The official Annual Report stated:

Dr. Oosterhuis, who was Medical Superintendent, proved to be unsuitable for the post. In April 1994 the Bishop, after much consultation and with the support of the DOG in Holland, which had recruited him, had to terminate his contract. Dr. Oosterhuis refused to leave until the Prime Minister's Office called him and told him to vacate the hospital premises. He left only at the beginning of December.

[Mission Doctors' resident permits were only valid as long as they were employed by a mission hospital - Editor.]

The unprecedented refusal of Dr. Oosterhuis to leave made it impossible for any doctor to work there. Dr. Meuwissen who had been the only doctor from April onwards had to go on leave in October1994. It was decided that doctors could only go back to Mantšonyane after Dr. Oosterhuis had left.

Dr. Paul Borgdorff kindly offered to interrupt his studies in Holland and return to Lesotho in September for six months. The DOG arranged for the necessary funds. We are grateful to Dr. Borgdorff, his wife and the DOG for the help. We are much indebted to them for the service which they so willingly gave.

Due to the crisis Mrs Khadi, the Matron decided not to continue her position at St. James'. We are grateful to her for all the work she has done over the last twelve years. She had been part and parcel of the growth and development of St. James' and we thank her very much for her contribution.

The above situation was obviously very difficult and unpleasant, but no official records are available. This sad episode should not be allowed to detract form the wonderful service, which the Dutch doctors provided from 1980.

Dr Liesbeth Meuwissen carried on with the PHC work until Dr. Paul Borgdorff took over from her in October 1994. After her two months leave Dr. Liesbeth and Dr. Paul returned to St. James' in mid-December to set about bringing the hospital back to normal, after being run by the nurses as a clinic, as best they could.

In 1993 outpatient attendance had fallen by 1000 and inpatients by 100. In 1994 outpatients recovered slightly though inpatients were down by a further 100. Remarkably, minor operations and deliveries remained constant during the traumatic year of 1994.

CHAPTER 11: TOWARDS THE MILLENNIUM.

Dr. Paul Borgdorff and Dr. Liesbeth Meuwissen faced a tremendous challenge when they returned to St. James' Hospital two weeks before Christmas, 1994.

When Liesbeth returned to Lesotho with Erik on 23rd September 1994, they brought with them two-month old son Peter Lerato (Love). A lot of love and care was required to reorganise the hospital completely as there had been no resident doctor in charge for three months, until Dr. Adekunle arrived in August from Nigeria and helped to get the hospital into swing again, until February.

The wards of the hospital were closed from 20th of February until 8th May to enable a fresh start to be made with regard to staffing. 'Mamotheo Lepheana was appointed Matron in January so that she could be involved in all new appointments. The outstation clinics had remained fully open throughout the difficult period.

Dr. Liesbeth wrote after her return:

We are very happy to be back and received a warm welcome from the staff. We were happy that the atmosphere was really good.

In spite of recent difficulties, we have kept all the clinic staff and some of the hospital staff have been reappointed, so there are still some people familiar with the hospital routine. 'Me Lepheana has done a very impressive job over the last few months to keep the hospital going. She introduced the new staff to their posts and the business has continued of serving the local communities well. During the last few months the hospital has functioned as a large Health Centre, seeing outpatients, delivering babies and continuing with primary health care. St. James' is now functioning as a normal hospital and we are quite busy.

In December 1994 Mrs Claurina Sixishe completed a record 16 years as bookkeeper/ secretary.

The female ward had been re-roofed and renovated with the help of the Reformed Church of Bilthoven, the Netherlands.

In October 1995 a third doctor, Theo Taakens joined Dr. Liesbeth and Dr. Adekunle. Dr. Theo came for three months and was sponsored by the 'Foundation Netherlands-Lesotho'.

When new staff were recruited a professional builder, Mr. Matlanyane, was appointed Head of the Maintenance Department. He soon set about repairs and renovations throughout the hospital. Ellen Scout became PHC Coordinator and Mr. Lebohang was taken on as Car Mechanic. For the first time in its history St. James' Hospital was well staffed with qualified midwives, as well at all the clinics.

At the end of 1995 Dr. Theo Taakens completed his three months service. He so liked the place that he promised to return in June of the next year and stay for three years. Dr. Henk Boerma, his wife, Saskia and their son, Jesse, aged two years, arrived through DOG of the Netherlands on a three year contract.

In February 1996 Mr. Job van Melle, the Director of the DOG visited the hospital personally. (the DOG had been responsible for sending doctors via their church related organisation for some twelve years and he wanted to see for himself the marvellous work these doctors were involved in.)

Saskia Boerma, whose Sesotho name was 'Mathabo (Mother of Joy) started a Pre- School Group in the hospital compound for the children of the staff, which was known as the 'Mathabo Pre-School.

[Some confusion arose later as the first doctor's wife to live at St. James' was also called `Mathabo, but she only taught Nurse Aids - Editor].

There were very limited schooling facilities like this in the area and this was one of the problems in attracting nurses to the hospital. Many people, from the surrounding, area applied for their children to join the 'Pre- School' so there were often 50 children in the class!

In March 1996, eight of the nurses received two weeks training in AIDS counselling and a poultry farm with 60 chickens was started.

In August 1996 Dr. Liesbeth wrote in her last report before returning to the Netherlands:

The hospital is functioning very well. We are busy and the atmosphere is very good. We have attracted many more nursing sisters and the hospital and clinics are now properly staffed.

At the end of June I ended my work at the hospital and handed over to Dr. Henk Boerma as Medical Superintendent. This left July for sorting out administrative matters and writing the Annual Report. I am also available for any advice and support needed by the new management.

Dr.Theo Taakens re-joined us in mid–June and has taken over as Director of the PHC work. These two doctors together with the Matron make up a strong team, who will work well with the staff for the improvement of the hospital and the benefit of the patients.

Dr Boerma wrote in his first letter:

Winter is holding Lesotho in its grip, with freezing nights and sunny days. People are harvesting the maize crop in abundance after poor harvests for several years. Maize (Poone) is the most important crop for most of the people and is the staple diet.

To give you an idea of the challenge we face I would like to share the story of one of our teenage patients. Lebohang is fourteen years old and lives with her grandparents not far from the hospital. His grandfather is not very well. Lebohang and his brother have looked after the sheep for many years. Lebohang has hardly ever seen a school from the inside. On the day we met he had had a dreadful accident. His brother had dislodged a big rock, which fell on Lebohang and broke his leg and crushed his foot. When brought to the hospital from the village he was afraid of things to come and on the verge of tears. Under anaesthetic his

wounds were cleaned and a pin bored through the heel so that the position of the fracture was good. His foot was badly damaged with multiple fractures. While we waited, counting the days, to see if the foot would mend properly, he received not a single visitor, despite several messages to the grandparents. His foot failed to heal properly and we took him to the hospital in Maseru. We followed him up on our visits to Maseru and he gradually improved. During all this time there was no sign of his parents. A message was finally got to his mother after about five weeks. When we last saw Lebohang he had been discharged, walking on crutches, his leg supported by a plaster. I wonder if I will see him again? Will he be able to walk properly? What will be his future?

By July the pre-school run by Saskia Boerma and helped by Lucia Kolotsane had 21 children from the staff and community. They had a mid-winter break and Saskia prepared a project proposal to encourage support for the school. In the meantime a parent committee had been formed and met to discuss the running of the school and to identify its needs. One outstanding need was for training teachers in our area. The idea was for the `Mathabo School to be a training centre to help other schools in the area to improve their standards. The pre-school started in the Training Hall of the hospital. Due to the need for this venue to be used for other training courses the old original prefabricated staff house became the home of the Pre-school and has continued as such.

The previous year's accounts had been audited and it was possible to set aside money for the replacement of vehicles. The Land-Rover Ambulance had served for eight years on rough roads and was no longer reliable.

In 1996 the Government of Lesotho restarted a supplementary feeding programme throughout the country. A co-ordinator for this important project, aimed to alleviate malnutrition in children, was attached to St. James'. Even grandfathers with donkeys came to collect the food!

It was, however, disappointing that the Government failed to honour the 'Memorandum of Understanding' signed in April 1995, to pay the full salaries of all professional hospital staff. In fact payments were reduced by £10 000 and promises to back date full pay were continually delayed. It was therefore very encouraging that the Royal Airforce in the UK agreed to pay a handsome annual grant of £10 000 per annum for four years through USPG to help the hospital to balance its books

On 2nd February 1997 a serious accident happened to Dr Henk, Saskia and Jesse Boerma.. Their vehicle was forced off the Mountain Road. Henk and Saskia sustained only minor injuries, but their son, Jesse, unfortunately, had a serious head injury and had to be taken to the Hydromed Hospital in Bloemfontein in the Orange Free State. When he was out of coma he had to be flown back to the Netherlands and of course his parents accompanied him. Thus the hospital was suddenly deprived of the services of Medical Superintendent and leader of the Pre-school. Dr Theo was therefore left once more with the difficult task of caring for both the hospital and the PHC Programme. Dr Theo did receive help both from Dr. Riches from Scotland and a Bulgarian doctor who came and helped for a month.

From July to November Dr. Khamar Abbasi from Pakistan came and rendered much needed assistance.

In June a new Laboratory was built and fully equipped by the Irish Government and two houses were started to accommodate the laboratory staff.

In September 'Me Lepheana left after two years and eight months as Matron. She had played no small part in the reorganisation of the hospital, but she was not immediately replaced.

Five new nurse's houses were built in 1997 with finances from the parish of Tilshead, Salisbury, UK, and the Pre-school continued to do well under L. Kolotsane, who had been trained by Saskia Boerma. In December, three children 'graduated' from the Pre-school, with due ceremony, organised by the parent's committee. The children danced and sang in the traditional Sesotho way. They were easily recognised by their special outfits and were ready now to continue their schooling in the local Primary Schools in the area, with great advantage.

In February 1998 the second woman doctor to give notable service to St. James' arrived. Dr. Simone Jaarsma was accompanied by her husband, Rob Van Acker and their son Sjoerd. Simone was sent by the DOG to be the 23rd doctor to work at the hospital and to become the 17th Medical Superintendent; she was to steer the hospital into the 21st century in a most capable way. Simone, although a Dutch Protestant, had grown up in Northern Italy, but trained in the Netherlands as a doctor. Rob, a designer by profession, was a Dutch Roman Catholic. Until the previous year they had been serving at a Mission Hospital in Uganda, but had to leave because of local unrest and fighting. Rob, as well as looking after their son, was eventually to be appointed Technical Adviser to keep an eye on equipment at the hospital and also in the outlying clinics as well as helping to produce the Annual Report.

It was good to have someone in charge of the hospital, which allowed Dr. Theo to concentrate his energies on the PHC. Talking to Colin Cockshaw from USPG, Dr Theo was concerned about many conditions going untreated or for which recourse was made to Traditional Healers. He did not consider working alongside Traditional Healers as a problem, provided they realised their limitations and knew when referral to the hospital or clinic was essential. He was also concerned that he rarely saw malnutrition in children and feared that poor families could not find the fees

On 1st April 1998 Dr. Tonny Mwabury joined the hospital staff from Tanzania, which meant for the first time in its history there were three doctors at Mantšonyane. As the second African doctor to serve at St. James', he recounted his experience and thoughts, after his first twelve months:

I find working in the remote mountains of Lesotho, both challenging and enriching, in that one is faced daily with extremely serious and potentially fatal, situations, needing speedy reactions and brain storming; it keeps one fully occupied.

St. James' Hospital, like all rural hospitals in Lesotho, has as common cases; assault, rape, tuberculosis (which could be AIDS related), sexually transmitted diseases together with ante-natal and post-natal complications.

Assault is quite common, principally by the 'molamu' (traditonal Basotho stick). People are often beaten by each other, particularly after getting drunk. This leads to fractured skulls, hands and legs. Being a patriarchial society, women are often beaten by men and are often so shy or afraid that they do not complain.

Sexual abuse is increasingly a worrying issue. 'Peto ea mosali'(rape) is common with even five year old children being abused by their relatives, 'Balisana' (Shepherd boys) easily side–track women along mountain paths and rape them. Despite appeals for these victims to seek urgent medical attention, they often appear at the hospital days after, which makes medical evidence for criminal charges more difficult.

Poverty plays a major part in the Mantšonyane HSA. Only about 15% have waged employment with the remainder struggling to survive on temporary unskilled jobs. They also depend largely on subsistence agriculture, which is unreliable due to erratic climate. Only 10% of households produce enough to feed themselves. There is insufficient grass because of overgrazing and much land is monopolised by some of the Barena (chiefs). Thus with many living below the poverty line or barely existing, one can hardly expect to have a healthy immune system and consequently they have poor resistance to disease.

[We were pleased to note a marked improvement in the nutrition of the school children on our visit in April 1999, compared with thirty years ago! – Editor]

The adult male records are unimpressive due to common and ever increasing sexually transmitted disease (STD), which is often accompanied by tuberculosis. Also, the social and economic situation of Lesotho has changed for the worse with the construction of dams for harnessing water at Katse and Mohale. The financial status of those working on the dams has improved a little, but promiscuity is a problem, while idle young ladies think that it is an opportunity to make more money by selling their bodies, only to end up with STD, particularly AIDS.

The infant and maternal mortality rates give rise to concern due to insufficient education of expectant mothers and irregular attendance at ante- natal clinics, or not attending at all. It is tragic, when some of them arrive at hospital with severe complications when their condition is very difficult to help.

Last, but not least, is the powerful influence exerted by the 'Nkhono', (Grandmother) or 'Mohoehali' (the man's mother-in-law) in the Sesotho traditional set-up in the homes.

[The first baby is usually delivered under the supervision of the woman's own mother, although the child is named by the Father's parents- Editor}.

Traditional influence often determines whether the young mother should go to hospital for delivery, the decision to stop breast-feeding or to continue having children, even if the woman's body is failing. A great deal of health education is required in projecting better health, as well as social attention and care by the health staff. If patients are looked down on, not talked down to politely or shouted at, or examined with gloves on, this breaks down their morale. Therefore sensitisation of hospital staff remains a 'sine qua non' for good service. Their participation in seminars and workshops plays no small part in improving patient care. I would also recommend the hospital not to lose sight of the need for continual updating of clinical skills through the many agencies who offer this facility.

It is my prayer for all donors supporting this hospital that they may continue their great support which is highly appreciated.

I would like to remind staff that we should not forget the primary goal of ' Care for patients'.

I would also like to pray that we live each day of our lives the way we would if Christ himself were here with us. I bear my testimony, that the strength I have, is to dedicate myself with a strong commitment to those who are in need, doing missionary work when required. I bear this testimony in Christ's name, who was resurrected on the third day. Amen.

Dr. Tonny gives us a frank assessment of the more problematic health problems which most doctors only mention in passing or do not mention. It is good that an African doctor has remedied this situation in giving a heartfelt and realistic presentation with compassionate insight and advice to all involved in the work of a mission hospital. Dr. Tonny's remarks and sincere prayers are those of a Christian doctor in the face of many and great difficulties he has encountered first hand. He obviously cares deeply for the minds and spirits of his patients as well as their bodies. His words are of value to all, who work at St. James' or are involved in medical missionary work elsewhere. His highlighting of the less glamorous aspects of the work and the hidden needs of the staff present a challenge to all donors of the hospital to respond to these needs and not only the more appealing special projects. The on-going work of running the hospital and caring for the staff remains a most important one and we are grateful for Dr. Tonny drawing attention to them.

At the same time as Dr. Tonny Mwabury gave his account of the work Dr. Simone Jaarsma wrote:

One could be very pessimistic about life in general in Lesotho. But it is inevitable that working in a hospital exposes one to a lot of society's problems. The good things are not often seen in the hospital. Also because our HSA is so inaccessible it is hard for us to know how the average Basotho experience life. One thing that sticks in my mind is this year's summer, which was good in Mantšonyane. We had a lot of rain, so most crops grew well. It was a feast to see a village community harvesting an acre of wheat within an hour, all by hand. The young men cut the wheat with sickles, the stems were collected by the women, who carried them to a dry place. There the old experienced men stacked six-foot high heaps, while other men made binding ropes from grass. Everywhere you could see scattered golden heaps waiting to be threshed, when they were dry. This year the stems were long enough to be used for thatching the houses. After their work the workers had lunch together on the land and everyone took their share home.

This year the hospital has been able to buy a new ambulance which can be used to replace the seven year old 'Mahongkong' which was giving more and more mechanical problems. The new vehicle can be used for the transport of patients and goods and has been named 'Pere e Tšoeu' (White horse) because of its powerful engine and modern appearance. We are grateful to the supporters who made this purchase possible.

Several new nursing sisters were found in 1998 and from October Mr. Matthews Manohar was appointed Hospital Administrator and a medical student from the Netherlands, Brechtje, came to help for three months.

When Dr. Simone went on Maternity leave early in 1999, St. James' obtained a temporary replacement by another Dutch doctor, Cees Sluimer and Gavin Wooldridge, a medical student from the UK, helped in all departments.

Before she went on leave, Dr. Simone wrote about her experience with AIDS., which had been a progressive problem over the previous eight years in the Maloti.

AIDS is affecting more and more people. Unlike other African countries, where diarrhoea is the most common symptom, we often see a combination of recurrent or chronic respiratory infections and weight loss. It is surprising how many ways this syndrome can show itself. In my first week at St. James' last year I admitted a well fed healthy looking lady, aged 34 years who was unconscious. She had a very low blood sugar, which was responsible for her coma. She improved within an hour with intravenous glucose and I tried to find out the reason for her condition. She could have died if she had been working alone in the fields. She was not a diabetic on insulin or other medications, which could have lowered her blood sugar. She had not been fasting and had been feeling well until just an hour and a half before she became unconscious. We sent off blood samples to Maseru for more investigations and told her what to do if she felt weakness, sweating or shivering. The lady, who had two young children, was discharged. One month later we saw her in outpatients. At first I failed to recognise her as she had lost a lot of weight and had a terrible cough. We discussed with her the possibility of her being HIV positive and she agreed to be tested. The result of her test was unfortunately positive. After the cough had settled, many episodes of different complaints followed and just four months after her first admission, the poor woman died an hour after she had been readmitted complaining of general weakness.

Of course not all HIV positive patients develop full blown AIDS which leads to such an abrupt death. Many patients have dependent children and for whom carers have to be found if their parents die. AIDS is still a very taboo subject which makes it difficult for our counsellors to ask about subjects like: 'Who can take care of your children after your death? 'How are you protecting your partner?' Usually patients know from what they are suffering but tell no one else! This is because they fear that they will be neglected if their partner or other relatives find out. Consequently they often die very lonely in Lesotho - alone with their secret disease.

There is much work to be done in this field, both on the preventive side and in the care and support of infected people. Our AIDS Department at St. James,' works in many different fields besides counselling and testing. The Mantšonyane AIDS Prevention Programme sponsored by 'Angli-CORD (the Australian Anglicans Co-operating in Overseas Relief and Development). The idea is to develop a two -year project of R360 000, which is geared towards home based care and AIDS support groups in the villages. Education and counselling services are to be the main thrust of the project, which has also been helped by the Lesotho National Bank, Canada Fund and private donors.

St. James' Hospital gave birth to a new 'baby' in May 1998 - a Social Work Department. It is very small at the moment with just one member of staff, Ntate Mosiuoa Scout, a social worker.

He introduced himself and his new work as follows:

St. James' Hospital is growing from strength to strength these days and this new department is a positive sign of this. Yes it might be small with just me so far, but it is a first step forward. The new 'baby' is vital to our hospital, which serves some of the remotest areas of our beloved 'Kingdom in the Sky'. Lesotho was caught up in urbanisation, which influenced the rural to urban influx. Taxes were imposed and men were forced to go and work in the mines and factories of South Africa. This meant that rural poverty soared with the diminishing of arable land, very low levels of living and poor access to health services. Mantšonyane is a big part of this poverty stricken rural society and is full of social problems. Social work focuses on the interaction of people with their environment and is concerned with a diversity of field medicine, psychiatry, industry and the police to mention but a few. Since the department opened the most common cases handled are old age, destitution, problems with paying hospital fees, alcohol abuse, marital and family disputes and foster cases.

An eighteen-month old girl was recently admitted to the hospital with severe malnutrition. Her mother had died a year ago and the child left in the custody of a very old and poor grandfather, who loved her a lot but could hardly afford to feed himself, let alone the baby. The father was working as a cowherd in a distant village and had not visited the child when informed she was in hospital. On investigation I found that the father's sister in Maseru District was a very willing person to care for her and good facilities for upbringing were available in that area. This was agreed by the grandfather. After two months in hospital the little girl had improved very much and started to play and crawl. Once the doctors told me she was ready for discharge the problems really started. Suddenly the grandfather did not agree with the proposed solution. The other family members, who had never visited the child in hospital, started to get involved. There were also scandalous rumours spread around that the hospital was selling babies and children! The relatives decided that the child should be kept in hospital so that they could visit her once in a while! We could not agree to this proposal and considered it unhealthy to hospitalise a young child and damaging to her emotionally, socially and physically. I was back to square one and the whole process of finding suitable foster parents started again.

The grandfather became more co-operative. This time I managed to involve the father of the child and finally it was agreed to bring her up under the foster care of the father's sister in Maseru. A formal agreement was signed by the foster mother, the doctor, one witness and myself. Copies of the agreement were given to the chief, the local court and the senior social worker to whom the child was referred for surveillance. You will be pleased to know that the child is doing well and the grandfather has visited her once in Maseru.

‚Dr. Simone returned to St. James' with her lovely baby girl, Luna. She reported that; . **At the end of 1998 the hospital staff had met to reflect on and evaluate the year, thanking donors for their faith in us and their continuous support. We have also been looking forwards to 1999 and we have expressed intentions to improve in our weak points and have made new plans. Of course we have prayed to be assisted in spiritual, professional and financial ways, to be able to continue the work we are doing into the new millennium!**

In June 1999 Dr. Simone reported further about several celebrations:

On the 23rd of April 1999 we were visited by a group of 15 supporters from the Lesotho Diocesan Association in the UK. Dr. Ken Luckman and his wife, Hazel, stayed for two more days at St. James'. Dr Ken was the first Medical Superintendent who started this hospital from scratch. For me it was interesting to hear how the hospital started and I have enjoyed their visit very much. I have realised that many things have changed over the years, much has matured, but the growth of the hospital and its complexity have also grown; more staff, equipment, money and management. Also, the expectations of both staff and the HSA population have grown. This means that health service per patient has become more expensive and we rely more than ever on your support.

The 30th of April was the official opening of the new Mortuary by Mr.Tom Wright of the Irish Consul, as it was donated by Irish Aid from the Republic of Ireland. Bishop Andrew Duma, soon to retire on health grounds, blessed the new building.

The old mortuary was literally a 'big fridge' standing under an improvised roof with a capacity for twelve bodies. It had had to cope not only with those who died in hospital, but also in the whole community. Bodies have often to be kept until all the relatives have been informed and are able to attend for the funeral. This can take a week or more, especially with men working away from home. The relatives pay a small fee for this service. The new mortuary is a more spacious building and can accommodate twenty bodies. There is also an attached room and a covered stoep or verandah for waiting relatives. Appreciation was expressed for this essential new facility and the times were recalled when there was just a small rondavel to serve as a mortuary.

On the 20th of May 1999 was the official farewell to Dr. Theo Taakens, who left after serving St. James' for over three years. The speeches praised his work and commitment and the staff shared their gratitude and friendship with dances and songs. His work had not always been easy. For twelve months he worked without a permanent colleague and had to cope with many management tasks alone. His major achievement was a firm consolidation of the PHC work with its clinics. Dr. Theo has returned to the Netherlands where he is to specialise in gynaecology.

Dr. Theo was succeeded by a Nigerian doctor, Oladeji Falodun, (the third African doctor to serve at St. James'). He was to work mainly in the hospital while Dr. Simone took charge of the PHC Programme in co-operation with the co-ordinator 'Me Ellen Scout, wife of the social worker.

Dr Oladeji Falodun, after ten months at the hospital, wrote:

I am a Nigerian born medical graduate of the College of Medicine, University of Ibadan. I completed my internship training at the Teaching Hospital of the same university almost six years ago. I practised at several hospitals in Nigeria before proceeding to Lesotho. I am married and a committed Christian. I arrived in Lesotho in the middle of 1998 and since then I've practised at various clinics and hospitals. I was a locum medical officer at Maseru Private Hospital before I joined St. James' Hospital in June 1999.

Mantšonyane is a fairly remote place and the problem of communication was like a big monster staring me in the face on my arrival. The roads are poor. However, the cordial atmosphere within the hospital premises made adjustment easier.

St. James' Hospital does have a good future if there is adequate financial support from donors. Also improved financial involvement from the Government of Lesotho will definitely assist in reducing patients' fees, improving hospital attendance and get medical care within the reach of this very poor mountainous region of Lesotho, which is itself also a poor country.

The PHC activities of the hospital are still looking for support. The hospital equipment needs regular servicing, The hospital vehicles need replacement because of the deplorable condition of some of the roads.

The Bible in Ecclesiastes says : 'Money answereth all things.' I believe with good financial support the hospital will go a long way in meeting the needs of this poor community.

After completing her first year as Matron, Ntšiuoa Sello, wrote:

The Lord has been making it possible for me to carry on with my duties with the active support of Dr. Simone in particular and other members of the hospital management. The staff also have been very supportive and I have learnt a lot. The hospital management team and the board of the hospital had decided that I follow a course in Nursing Management in Botswana. The course was supposed to have started in April. However the course did not take off due to some management problems of the institution. I am still trying to find another place that offers such a course. The fact is, much as there are a lot of things to be learned on the job, there is still a dire need to acquire further skills through training.

The hospital staff has been somewhat steady the whole of last year with only one or two resignations. In general, staff are staying relatively longer which is good for continuity of care. With the bed-occupancy rate of only 33% for the last year we have in mind to carry out a mini survey to find out what issues surround the low utilisation rate of beds.

We have recently carried out a survey on staff interests, especially in the Nursing department in terms of where each one can utilise their skills to produce maximum results. The response was really amazing as we did it in the form of scheduled interviews. We are continuing with the analysis and I believe when the strategies are in place, we will have an improved service delivery. I believe in general we have a great potential. The staff is dedicated and keen on employing ways to improve the effectiveness and efficiency of the hospital. I believe there should ways to invest in the human resources of the hospital in terms of training for all the staff, including the management. Where there is a will, there is a way.

I'm sure God will see us through as He has His best interests vested in this hospital and in the community it serves.

In 1999, with donor support of the Lesotho-Durham Link, the staff houses were refurbished with basic furniture. A major concern during 1999 was that donor support for the PHC Programme ceased and reduced the money available for training purposes. Another concern was that the AIDS programme lacked a co-ordinator and only half the funds for this were utilised.

At the end of October 1999 Dr. Simone wrote an informative newsletter as follows:

It is still dry in Lesotho. People have ploughed, ready to sow and plant as soon as the rain starts. But until now the rain doesn't seem to be ready for Lesotho. Springs are becoming dry and the rivers are drying up. With insufficient water to wash the hands regularly, not to mention the rest of the body, we are seeing quite a number of people with gastro-enteritis together with skin and eye diseases.

At the hospital herd boys have been stuffing stones into the supply pipes between the spring and the tank to try and get water for their cattle. Part of the system needs to be rebuilt. Our other water supply needs a new underground tank, which our water engineer will tackle on his return. At present we have only running tap water for the houses for a few hours every other day. The rest of the time we have to collect water from a water point in the compound. We economise on water use by washing the babies first, then the mothers and then the nappies and finally use the waste-water to flush the toilets. We wash our hands with then a cup of water. We use polythene gloves to examine patients.

In October King Letsie III asked for prayers for rain. A severe dust storm damaged many houses though the hospital was not damaged, but still no rain! The traditional practice of grass burning to encourage the growth of a quick bite for the animals stimulates soil erosion.

Our new sophisticated laboratory is funded and staffed by Irish Aid. Martina Conion arrived in April 1999 to work in the laboratory for two years and lives in a smart house also built by Irish Aid. She is an Apso volunteer and writes a newsletter to the hospital staff and health centres:

"It is our continuing wish to develop our microbiology department into performing cultures and antibiotic sensitivities. This is important with respect to STD, which is otherwise treated blindly. A lot of resistant organisms are now showing up, due to proper full courses of antibiotics not being completed by patients. If we manage to begin this work we will require sufficient workload to sustain it, as experienced in other CHAL hospitals.

A big welcome back to 'Me Pheletso who has returned to work here having completed her studies in Ireland for her certificate in medical laboratory science. She is now working in the laboratory and Ben

Motjeane is now covering maternity leave in the Pharmacy/ X- ray department.

In July a group of volunteers from the Lesotho- Durham Link came to erect a playground for the children. Half the volunteers built the playground, while the others painted and decorated the new recreation, formerly used by the PHC (now in their new building). This new facility enables staff members to have tea breaks, play table tennis and watch satellite television. Previously the board- room had been used for staff recreational purposes.

Dr Simone's first newsletter in the year in the year 2000 said:

Thank you very much for the Christmas and New Year cards and also Christmas donations from many supporters. In Mantšonyane the jump into the New Year came without any 'millennium bug' problems. On Christmas Eve the staff went round the wards to sing and pray with the patients. As every year, small presents were given to the patients. After that we had drinks with the staff and most people went home to celebrate Christmas with their families. The hospital party, which is usually held on New Year's Eve, took place after the General Staff meeting back in November. All the staff from the hospital. health centres and Water Project, discussed different issues affecting the hospital. At the Cultural Night afterwards many different dishes were prepared, songs and dances were performed, people wore their national costumes and explanations were given. We had contributions from Ireland, the Netherlands, Nigeria and of course, Lesotho. It was good to see how many talents we have in the hospital community. During Christmas and New Year we usually see many patients with alcohol and violence related problems, but fortunately this year has been very quiet. We hope this is the start of a new trend.

Last October our ancient X-ray machine broke down and spare parts were unobtainable; so we are referring patients to other hospitals for X-ray, to come back to us for treatment. We eventually got hold of a second hand machine and think we have found a donor to replace this expensive piece of equipment, which is so essential. Rains eventually came in November and everything looks green and lush.

The annual report of April 1999 to March 2000 gives us more recent news:

The hospital received this year a lot of support from donors for general running costs and also for projects. All the staff houses have been supplied with new or rehabilitated solar systems for warm water. The incinerator and surrounding area have been rehabilitated and fenced.

Miss Karen Arnold, a medical student from the UK came to join us for two months.

A small girl of three years old was seen for the fifth time during the year in the out-patient department. Like the previous times the child was breathless, feverish and a productive cough. The diagnosis pneumonia was made again and treatment was started. After asking the mother what she did at home to prevent her child falling sick, she replied that she always put the child in the smoke of the fire as she thought that the warmest place of the house. After explaining to the mother that smoke is very irritative to the lungs and through that may be contributing to the recurrent severe chest infections, the mother and child went home. Since then we have not seen the little girl back with a chest infection.

In February 2000 Mr Matthews Monahar left after less than 18 months service as administrator.

It was not possible to fill the post of administrator until the 1st of July, when Mr. Ademola Aseperi began work. The last newsletter of 2000 provided the welcome news that Dr. Oladeji Falodun who left in May had been replaced by Dr. Roger Phanzu from the Democratic Republic of Congo in August 2000.

It was therefore good news to have three doctors again, at least until the end of April 2001, when Dr. Jaarsma left. Dr. Tonny Mwabury had agreed to take over the PHC as director, but unfortunately has resigned for personal reasons.

Therefore Dr. Phanzu remains the sole doctor having to cope with both the hospital and the clinics.

In July 2001, after almost a year at St James', he wrote as acting Medical Superintendent:

I graduated from Kinshasa in 1995 and worked in one of our hospitals in the Democratic Republic of Congo, before travelling to South Africa in 1997, where I hoped to find work until I was accepted here in Mantšonyane. It is difficult to express completely my first impressions as I am still trying to settle into my new position. The hospital is still relying a lot on donors because of the poverty of the population. The PHC is still running programmes needing support from donors. With the exception of the domestic and maintenance departments, it is difficult to keep people for long. I believe in giving doctors and nurses their needs in order to have a permanent team. Also, a stable income is needed to satisfy the hospital budget requirements. A lot can still be done in the PHC if the finances could be found.

CHAPTER 12: THE PRIMARY HEALTH CARE PROGRAMME.

'The Lord sent them out into every village.' (LK 10.1 CEV)

Having completed the general history of St James' Hospital, we devote a whole chapter to the development of a most exciting and vitally important aspect of the health care provided by the clinics in the Primary Health Care Programme, widely known as the ' PHC Programme'.

After an overview of the programme we will give more detailed accounts of the various clinics, their work and how they have developed over the last 40 years.

In August 1999 Dr. Simone Jaarsma commented in her annual report:

Curative services in the hospital are necessary but they hardly influence the health status of the community. Western health care and basic health principles (Hygiene, nutrition etc.) are not yet accepted and implemented among many of the households of the Mantšonyane Health Service Area (HSA)

The PHC Programme has two objectives:

The first is to bring curative and preventive health services nearer to the community through satellite clinics.

The second objective is to achieve in the long term, a healthier lifestyle, for which participation of the community and voluntary village Health Workers (VHWs) is essential.

The growth of clinics served by the hospital and the development of the PHC Programme have been quite a remarkable achievement, especially over the last 17 years, since the most helpful support from 1983 of the German church agency, the 'Evangelische Zentrallstell für Entwicklungshilfe' (EZE). This programme has produced far-reaching benefits to the whole area in making both curative and preventive services far more accessible to the Basotho of the area.

It had been a long term objective to do this right from the beginning of the medical work. As long ago as 1962, encouragement was given to these local communities to provide simple buildings. Before the hospital was opened, exploratory visits were made by Dr. Ken Luckman to enable regular visits to begin at Ha Mafa and in Ha Khomari in the remote Lesobeng valley.

Progress was slow and it was not until November 1969 that Dr. Nicholas Cohen was able to begin visiting these two mobile clinics (later called semi-permanent clinics) on horseback..

The Government Health Centre at Ha Marakabei was supervised and visited by a doctor from the hospital every week from July 1961 and in August 1970 Dr. Nicholas Cohen also took over the government clinic at Likalaneng. Both these clinics were accessible from the Mountain Road by Four-Wheel Drive.

The PHC Programme received fresh impetus in 1980 with the appointment of Dr. Walter Tjon- A-Ten as Medical Superintendent.

In March 1981 a Co-ordinator was appointed for the training of Village Health Workers (VHWs.) who were to become responsible for a key role in PHC together with Matron Veronica Khadi.

In July 1982 Under-Fives Clinic were begun at Ha Mafa and Likalaneng. The Marakabei Health Centre was taken over completely from the Lesotho Government by St. James' Hospital. Four years later, a new impressive Health Centre was built to replace the dilapidated original one.

By 1988 there were six permanent clinics with resident staff and two semi-permanent Clinics being visited and three Village Health Posts were being started. These efforts were in line with the National Lesotho Health Policy, which was something of a pioneering venture in Southern Africa and firmly based on the PHC concept and the Alma-Ata Declaration of 1978.

Thus St.James' became more and more the focus of health services in the Mantšonyane HSA, including both curative and preventive work and the promotion of Latrine Construction of which 108 were built in 1988, making the total of 422. Maternal and Child Health, immunisations, nutritional health education and control, of infectious diseases were all part of the programme. In addition the training of VHWs and Traditional Birth attendants were important too and were financed from UNI CEF. Courses were also arranged for the Traditional Healers, Chiefs and Teachers through help from the main donor of the PHC, the EZE. In 1994 the clinics were being visited by a team of doctor, Matron, Public Health Nurse and the Pharmacy Technician. Some clinics were only staffed by Nurse Assistants, who were very good.

In the Annual Report of 1995-1996 it was proudly stated that every Health Centre was well staffed with Midwives and Health Assistants for the environmental health and outreach activities. Mrs Eileen Scout (wife of the social worker), an experienced Health Educator was appointed as Co-ordinator of the PHC. She also joined the hospital management team of St. James' Hospital.

From January 1999 the PHC was being run without the valuable support of EZE, which had supported the Programme since 1983. This meant that the PHC had to be financed by the hospital budget. There were anxieties expressed concerning the repercussions for both the hospital and the PHC and great efforts were made to find a new donor for the PHC as soon as possible. Dr Theo Taakens was Director of the PHC Programme 1996-1999. Let him speak for himself:

The PHC is a department with its different small units scattered throughout the HSA. The advantage of being independent, is to run your own Centre or Clinic, close to the people you serve. The disadvantage is not having a doctor to back you up and of poor communication via a not very reliable two-way radio system. A lot has been achieved, although it

has not always been easy, since all efforts partly depend on the commitment of the local people.

The four A's are the big challenges:

ACCESSIBILITY: The Mantšonyane catchment area is among the remotest of the country. Essential health services have to be brought closer to the public by means of five Health Centres, two Permanent Clinics, and Village Health Posts.

AFFORDABILITY: The fees for registration and drugs are kept as low as possible. Health Education and all outreach activities are free of charge.

APPROPRIATE: There is a referral system and a monthly supervisory visit for consultation and support. Home based care is available for emergencies; an ambulance service is available.

ACCEPTABILITY OF HEALTH CARE: A lot of effort is put into Health Education and explanation to the patients, especially about Family Planning. Key figures of the community are targeted to help to deliver health messages. PHC means going for the 'basics first, essential needs and prevention. It was designed to minimise the occurrence of preventable diseases and to improve the health status of the population in general. That is why water and sanitation has always been a big part of our programme and our water project such a success.

In June 1998 our PHC staff moved from a small office to the new PHC Building with five offices, a main hall and storage space. Before, the U/5s Clinic, ante-natal check-ups and counselling for HIV positive clients were done in the same room with other staff attending or walking in and out. The corridor and the neighbouring chapel have all kinds of secrets of patients taken there for privacy!

Since May 1998 our Social Worker has helped the PHC to recognise all kinds of social problems affecting health. At first he joined the doctor's visits to the Health Centres to make the staff more aware and help them to support these kinds of patients. The Health Assistants especially have been sensitised to the fact that environmental health can be very unsociable as well; for example the dumping of solid waste from one family in front of the rondavel of another.

Home-based care is one of the items developed under the influence of the AIDS Programme. A number of HIV-positive patients can be treated very well at home for opportunistic infections they acquire. It is always amazing to experience the unbelief of patients when they are informed of their HIV-status, but even more when infected with the very severe *Tuberculosis bacillus*, when you tell them they can be treated for it. After at least 14 days of hospital treatment TB patients can often go home and have their medicine daily supervised by a VHW or a reliable neighbour or relative. This has reduced the cost of admissions and makes the patient feel more a part of the community. The results have proved encouraging and compliance with treatment good. As PHC Director, I like going out to communities very much, riding on horseback and seeing patients in their homes. To see and experience how they live, their lifestyle and friendly attitude towards the 'ngaka ea sekhooa' (white doctor) and traditional health beliefs. They paint my days. Drinking at times the local brew, not thinking too much about hygiene or the level of fermentation. A lot of goodwill is received and most of the time it is well appreciated.

Constantly we need to go back to 'basics' How we love to do our heroic western sophisticated medicine, but we must start with the 'basics'- to sensitise, make aware and educate in the terminology of the people is important- from mother and child care, immunisation, communicable diseases, essential drugs and the treatment of minor illnesses to water and sanitation, construction of water systems and latrines. Training is the cornerstone of this work and outreach activities are the necessary follow up

Everybody is invited to have a taste of this work! Your support to keep us and our cars going over the tracks in this beautiful landscape is highly appreciated and necessary. On behalf of the Basotho people, we thank you in the hope of your continued interest and support.

We now describe the development of the network of individual clinics which are scattered throughout the Mantšonyane HSA served by the PHC Programme of St. James' Mission Hospital. Those who have supported special projects over the years will see how their efforts have benefited these isolated communities.

HA MARAKABEI HEALTH CENTRE.

Ha Marakabei Health Centre is situated 15 miles from St. James' Hospital, about three miles from the bridge over the Senqunyane River. The HC was established by the Basutoland Government in the mid 1950's and consisted of corrugated iron buildings for the clinic and resident staff nurses. Further corrugated iron buildings were later added for deliveries, Health Assistant and Mortuary. From July 1961, the doctor from Mantšonyane took over the responsibility of supervising the HC and visited weekly on Wednesdays and used to see anything up to 100 patients. He was also responsible for carrying out Post-mortem examinations on behalf of the government and even exhumations. This latter part of the work was very time consuming and necessitated visits to Maseru to give evidence in court. It is not surprising that after some years, this aspect of the work was relinquished so as to concentrate on patient care. There were always difficulties about the adequate supplies of medicines from the government and so in July 1982 the HC was completely taken over by St. James' Hospital from the Lesotho Government. Plans were set in motion to build an entirely new modern HC to replace the dilapidated old one. A Dutch Roman Catholic organisation, CEBEMO (Stichting

Nederland-Lesotho), and the EEC offered to sponsor the new HC, which took four years to build.

The new Health Centre was opened on 15th March 1986 and was blessed by the Bishop Donald Nestor, assistant bishop of the diocese and a 'Mokete' was held.

The catchment area of this HC is very extensive and the new building needed to cater for curative and preventive care and also for deliveries of a vast number of patients. The new facilities included a consulting room, a training U5 hall, a dispensary, a two-bedded labour ward, a two-bedded maternity ward and a waiting mothers' lodge. There were also three staff houses for the four resident nurses and a shelter for the night watchman and horses. Solar energy was utilised for light, hot water and water pump. A Nursing Sister was in charge and a whole PHC supportive team worked both at the HC and in the surrounding communities.

Since September 1985 the nurses from the HC have paid monthly visits to Ha Mpeli which is three hours' horse-ride away along a very difficult track, for U/5s and ante- natal clinics. The VHP is supervised locally by the VHW s and is very active and well attended. In 1989 the VHP was temporarily suspended due to lack of local co-operation but was reopened in the following year and monthly visits from the HC recommenced.

Marakabei HC continues as the busiest one of the HSA with an average total of 2,500 attendances a year. It is a model HC of which the Anglican Church of Lesotho and St. James' can justly be proud.

HA LEPHOI HEALTH CENTRE.

Ha Lephoi Health Centre lies 28 miles from St. James' Hospital in the remote Lesobeng valley. It used to take four to five hours along a rough road by Four-Wheel Drive when work was started there in 1983 with a semi-permanent and U/5s clinic. Two rivers need to be negotiated and during heavy rains it is sometimes impossible to get there, in spite of improvement in the road since 1990, which has shortened the journey to two and a half hours.

The HC is owned by the Anglican Church of Lesotho ('Kereke ea Chache'), the Sesotho name which derives from the early missionaries who spoke about 'the Church', presumably with a rather sophisticated accent! St James' Hospital has of course been responsible for staffing and supplies from the beginning, 28 years ago.

In May 1985 a permanent clinic was established by funds from the EZE in Bonn, Germany. It consisted of a rondavel attached to a three- roomed building, which served as a kitchen, store, lecture-room, and accommodation for one PHC Motivator. There was a separate building for the Nurse and a small stable for horses. The original staff consisted of 'Me Mamotheo Lepheana as Nurse Clinician in charge, two PHC Motivators, a ward attendant and a maintenance man This clinic became one of the busiest in the HSA. In June 1986 a course for teachers was held at the clinic.

In 1992 an impressive new HC began to be built with further help from the EZE which had already been a vital supporter for nine years.

In 1993 the clinic became the important base for the Lesobeng Spring Protection Project, backed by welcome donations from CEBEMO and Irish Aid.

The work was very competently organised by Erik van der Giesson, husband of Dr. Liebeth Meuvissen and a qualified water engineer. Construction began in earnest in February 1994 with the protection of nine springs and 82 springs had been protected by 1999, serving 4000 Basotho with clean safe drinking water in their villages. The villagers did most of the work themselves. Two people were selected from each village and trained as 'Water Minders' to maintain the water gravity systems. The skilled work involved was carried out by four masons trained by Village Water Supply, Lesotho. As a result each villager was enabled to collect 30 litres of clean water a day from a tap within 160 yards from their dwelling. A Water Committee in each village collects the 'seabo', a contribution towards the maintenance fund from each household in the village.

In 1994 Ha Lephoi clinic became very difficult to reach again as the road had deteriorated badly and was very poor, especially in the rainy season. However the doctor from St. James' continued monthly visits by use of the Lesotho Flying Doctor Service (LFDS) On the first of June 1996 after four years of difficult work, the clinic was re-opened as a full Health Centre. The new building was beautiful with two excellent Delivery Rooms and eight beds for short stays, a room for health education, and a guestroom. The new HC became the first proper medical centre for the area, serving about 14 000 Basotho with daily facilities. The old clinic was converted into a Waiting Mother's Lodge. World AIDS Day was held at Ha Lephoi HC in December 1997.

The 1996-1998 reported staff difficulties and changes and a new Nurse in charge was being sought. Even so attendances were maintained although preventive activities were reduced.

In 1998 Colin Cockshaw from USPG visited the HC and gave the following account of his visit to supporters:

Steady numbers arrived throughout the morning from the surrounding villages, many on foot, some on horseback. Many of the women came in their Sunday best complete with stockings (although most had to ford a river to reach the HC) and umbrellas for protection from the sun. One lady had arrived the previous evening and given birth to a boy an hour before we arrived. More typically, however, Basotho men and women go everywhere clad in traditional blankets. Women often wear a woolly hat, which can be pulled down over their faces for extra weather protection, while men wear the Basotho straw hats. Dr. Jaarsma invited me to sit in on part of her clinic, so I was able to see something of local health problems at first hand. The patients included a

lady seeking birth control advice, a baby with chest infection, a man recovering form TB, but believed to be HIV positive, a young lady with an undiagnosed mental problem and a young man who had been injured in a fight. I gathered all these cases were quite common. The health worker at Ha Lephoi translated for Dr. Jaarsma and also dealt with some parts of the advice

On the return journey to Mantšonyane we brought in the pick-up a double bed belonging to a nurse returning to work at St, James' and lying on the bed was a retired school teacher from the village, who required some urgent difficult dental treatment.

In June 1999 Dr. Simone Jaarsma described a visit to Ha Lephoi HC and also to the clinic at Mont Martre RC Mission 38 miles from St. James'. It had been supervised by the hospital since 1987 when it was taken over from the LFDS after it had served the clinic for a year. Mont Martre is quite a busy clinic with about 1 500 attendances a year.

Dr. Simone says:

I am very much enjoying visits to the HCs, especially going to Mont Martre. We try to leave early. After a one and a half hours' drive through beautiful scenery, we arrive at Ha Lephoi and from there I continue by horse for another one and a half hours to reach Mont Martre Clinic. Sometimes there are only eight patients; other times more than twenty. After seeing the patients and talking and eating with the friendly nurses, I return to Ha Lephoi where I spend the night. The next day I see patients at the HC and discuss issues with the nurses and Health Assistants. Three hours west of Mont Martre, along a difficult track, a VHP at Ha Makara, is staffed by the nurses who provide U/5s and Ante-Natal care.

Mr. Dasharatha Nyaupane, a water engineer from the mountains of Nepal, took over the Lesobeng Water Project from Erik van der Giesson in July 1996. He gives us a further update of his three years in charge of the project:

The work in Lesobeng is very rewarding. People appreciate our work. I work with a nice team, which also feel responsibility for the project. At the moment, we have a project co-ordinator, that is me, a technical officer, a health assistant, a project assistant a driver and seven masons.

Although there are plenty of springs, when they are not properly protected, they become contaminated with surface water. This can lead to many health problems such as diarrhoea and Typhoid fever. Many still do not understand that there is a connection between diseases and contaminated water. We start by visiting and meeting with the whole community to explain health problems related to water and the responsibilities of the community and the project. A Village Water Committee, half of them women, receives training about different systems available, how they are constructed and managed. In addition hygiene issues and basic book- keeping for fund maintenance are covered. They also have to organise voluntary labour to help; only the masons are paid by the project. Villages usually choose a simple gravity system, which is easier to maintain in the future. Transport of materials has to be arranged, as Four-Wheel Drive cannot reach many of the villages. Donkeys are very useful for carrying cement bags. After a year, the village has become entirely responsible for the system. By September 2000 we will have finished the project in the Lesobeng valley and we will have covered the valley. Systems have been built for 132 villages since the beginning of the project, protecting about 300 springs, serving 17 000 people. From Lesobeng we plan to move on towards Methalaneng and Ha Popa, following the Senqunyane River. Knowledge gained at Lesobeng will be useful to us in working in the mountains of Lesotho, which are not unlike those of my home country, Nepal.

There have been recent difficulties with staffing of the HC with Nursing Sisters and Trained Nursing Assistants have been in charge and a new Health Assistant has been busy with community activities.

METHALANENG HEALTH CENTRE.

Methalaneng Health Centre is situated in the remote Methalaneng valley about twenty miles from St. James' Hospital. It takes about three hours by road to reach the HC which began originally as a clinic of the Lesotho Government in 1982, but had to be closed because of difficult of access.

In 1984, after the government re-opened the clinic, Dr. Jan Voskens began visiting on horseback once a month from St. James'; the road was not yet completed and a proposed airstrip was still on paper.

Then in March 1987 the clinic was re-opened yet again as by this time the airstrip had been completed next to the clinic. The Lesotho Flying Doctor service and St. James; Hospital agreed to supervise it jointly by air. The clinic could now be reached in ten minutes provided flying conditions were good. This was a vast improvement on a very rough ride by horse from the Hospital!

In 1990 the clinic became a Government Health Centre and included a delivery ward, dispensary, out-patients, and three staff houses. Sadly in 1992 the Health Centre lost its nurse and nurse assistant, but Maternity and Child Health services were continued by St, James' Hospital .In 1994 a Nurse Clinician, 'Me Paballo Thato, was appointed by the government and the HC returned to full operation.

Unfortunately in October 1997 there was a robbery at the HC and a month later, there was a serious crash of an aeroplane of the Mission Aviation Fellowship, just after take off. Sadly the pilot, a well-known Christian was killed. The HC once again, ceased to operate as such, but a team from St. James', consisting of a doctor, nurse PHC nurse pharmacy technician and a revenue collector, visited once a month by MAF plane for curative, U/5s and ante-natal services. About 60 patients usually attend.

In 1999 the HC was still only reachable by plane and a doctor and a nurse from St. James' were alternating visits with the LFDS every two weeks.

Dr. Simone reported:

The first time I went, was a freezing cold beautiful clear day in the middle of winter. More than 60 patients were waiting to be seen and there is no resident nurse at present. The nurse and I started to see them immediately because after four hours the pilot was due to collect us again. After a few hours I heard the plane, but there were so many patients still to be seen that we did not go outside to look. After half an hour, one of us went outside to see if there was enough time to see more patients, but discovered that there was no plane on the airstrip at all! At that moment there was a radio call to inform us that landing was impossible due to weather conditions and they would try again the next day! We finished the consultations when it was almost dark and very, very cold. There were no blankets or food anywhere and everybody had gone home. A little bit later we started to collect some scarce firewood and we found some anthracite. That night we tried to sleep around the fire made in the stove of one of the rooms of the abandoned nurse's house, eating some biscuits and telling each other stories. The next day we were delivered direct to Maseru for me to attend a meeting early that morning.

LIKALANENG HEALTH CENTRE

Likalaneng Health Centre, also owned by the Government of Lesotho is 28 miles down the Mountain Road from St. James' Hospital. Dr. Nicholas Cohen began visiting the clinic there in 1970 and doctors from St. James' continued to visit the clinic, which also gave U/5s services until 1983.

A new government clinic was built by August 1984, but was still not open after seven months. In fact it was not re-opened until 1985 when St. James' Hospital resumed visiting monthly.

In 1987 the annual attendance of patients at Likalaneng was 6 170 - the highest of all the clinics in the HSA for that year.

By 1993 the clinic was operating as a HC with a Nurse Clinician in charge, assisted by a Nurse Assistant.

In October 1996 the HC was officially closed by the Government as they were unable to replace the Nurse Clinician and only a Nurse Assistant and a night watchman remained. No supervisory visits were made from St. James'. The hospital offered several times to assist at least with Ante-natal services, but the offer was not taken up by the Government. However TB patients are referred from the government clinic at Mohale Dam to the hospital at Mantšonyane. The trained Nurse Assistant continued to hold U/5s and Ante-natal clinics on her own without medical supervision. After a year of being partly closed, a team from St. James' now attends monthly by MAF plane. The LFDS do likewise, so providing in all a fortnightly service. A VHP has been opened at Ha Korporala

HA POPA HEALTH CENTRE.

Ha Popa Health Centre is situated 17 ½ miles from St. James' Hospital, south of Auray RC Mission and clinic. This important HC serves the area between the Mantšonyane and Senqunyane Rivers. The access road is poor and the HC is one of the most isolated in the HSA and most probably also the poorest in Lesotho. The clinic began life as a VHP about 1980 and this became a semi-permanent clinic in 1983 under the care of the Anglican Church of Lesotho with St. James' Hospital responsible for staffing and supplies and was visited initially by the PHC staff on horseback. An U/5s clinic was soon begun

In January 1987 a Permanent Clinic was opened. The clinic was staffed by VHWs. and first visited by Dr. Jan Voskens by road with Four-Wheel Drive. At the end of 1991 work began to upgrade the clinic to a Health Centre with the financial support of the Lesotho-Durham Link, a most valuable direct link between the Anglican diocese of Lesotho and Durham, with an office in Maseru, efficiently managed by Dr. Peter Green. The EEC in Brussels and the Overseas Development Administration in the UK also gave their support to this most important project for some of the most needy Basotho of the country.

In May 1993 the new beautiful Health Centre of Ha Popa was officially opened, with a local 'mokete' attended by about 800 people. Appropriately, Joalane Mokeretla, a thirteen year old girl, who had been born in the original Village Health Post, cut the bandage across the entrance and led the way round the building as it was blessed by the bishop. Afterwards the bishop celebrated an open-air Mass.

The new HC consisted of a consulting room, a dressing room, a dispensary, a training room, a waiting room, a labour ward, and a maternity ward, which could accommodate four mothers and a waiting mother's lodge. A large lounge connected the clinic with a two bed-roomed staff house. At a later date, a smaller house was built, next to the stables, by the Lesotho Government through the Rural Clinics Maintenance programme.

Initially there was a trained Nurse Assistant in charge of the HC, but she was replaced in 1996 by a Nurse Midwife.

In 1998, the stables were converted into a larger Waiting Mother's Lodge and rondavels provided for the horses.

In 1999, it was thought that the HC was not being used as much as it might be. Although it had been built at the request of the local population of about 10 000 people, less than 200 patients a week were actually attending. The HC is fully staffed with six members. In view of its under-usage, it is a relatively expensive health care delivery facility. This is a pity, but many people in such a poor area, simply cannot afford the fairly modest fees charged. It is to be hoped that an agreement between the Government of Lesotho and CHAL can be reached, which will enable the Mission Hospitals which all belong to CHAL to use the same fee structure as the Government Hospitals. This might solve the burning financial problems of the local people as well as the HC, so that all the facilities will be fully used in the future.

However it is good to report that over 1000 patients have attended both for immunisations and the U/5s clinics for the last two or three years.

AURAY CLINIC.

Auray Clinic is the nearest to St. James' Hospital and only 4miles along the road to Lesobeng. The clinic is part of the Roman Catholic Mission at Ha Nyane. There has always been a friendly relationship with the Roman Mission and a most cordial co-operation with the Anglican hospital of St. James', right from the very first days in 1961.

The clinic was first opened in 1985 with a Nurse Assistant and a helper and doctors from St. James' have visited and supervised from the beginning. The clinic is only one small room as the nurse in charge actually lives at the Mission. In 1988 a double qualified Nurse/Midwife was appointed and the U/5s and Ante-Natal clinics began.

In 1997, a Nursing Sister, Bernadette Maseli took charge of the clinic and was still working there in 1999. Attendances have declined somewhat over the last ten years, but over 1000 a year attend for both U/5s and immunisation in addition to almost 1000 outpatients and ante- natal visits.

In the early days, the nurse from Auray, visited a VHP at Ha Mpeli and since 1993, she has been actively involved in developing a VHP at Madomaneng on the other side of the mountain range, in the direction of the Senqunyane River. It serves several large villages. The people built the walls of the clinic and helped the PHC staff to construct a protected spring, while St. James' roofed the clinic and provided doors, windows and glass. The land was provided gladly by the local chief. In 1996 there was some social unrest in the area, which hampered the work of the VHP. Auray Mission is quite involved in social work and hopefully will help to solve local problems at Madomaneng.

HA MAFA CLINIC.

Ha Mafa was in fact the very first village, only 12 miles from St. James' Hospital, to be seriously considered as a suitable place for an outstation clinic in the early '60s. Dr. Ken Luckman was often called to visit patients on horseback and was well received by the local chieftainess, Mofumahali Mampoi Matete. She was quite interested in the possibility of a clinic to serve her large village, which was the centre of the long established Lesotho Evangelical Church, founded by the Paris Evangelical Missionary Society, (PEMS) The people did actually start building a rondavel clinic, but progress was very slow indeed and it was not until November 1969, that Dr. Nicholas Cohen was able to commence a semi-permanent clinic. This involved half a day's horse riding which together with seeing the patients took a whole day. The local people's co-operation in building a permanent clinic was again very protracted and visits were discontinued after a few years until Dr. Walter Tjon-A-Ten started to visit again in October 1980.

A village Health post building was eventually commenced in July 1985 but the two rondavels were not ready for opening as a semi-permanent clinic until November 1987, when the Director of UNICF and the secretary of PHAL attended the long awaited ceremony. The clinic was the responsibility of the Anglican Church of Lesotho. It was staffed by a PHC Motivator, who in August 1998, went for training as a Nurse Assistant at the Scott Hospital, Morija. Her duties were taken over by another Trained Nursing Assistant and the clinic, visited monthly by a doctor from St. James'. The TNA held clinics five days a week, so providing the community with basic outpatient and preventive services, such as an U/5s clinic.

The clinic still consists of the two rondavels, constructed by the community, but improved in 1994 by the Rural Clinics maintenance programme, when ceilings were put in. The performance of the clinic has not increased over the past ten years and only about 500 patients attend per year. An Ante- Natal clinic operates when the doctor pays the monthly visit, while the U/5s clinic receives support from the PHC team.

There is a great need for the local water spring to be protected properly before this semi-permanent clinic can develop further as a proper permanent clinic.

In approaching 40 years, comparatively little progress has been achieved at Ha Mafa and it would be easy to give up efforts there. However with continued support of St. James' Hospital and the PHC team, it would be marvellous to celebrate the new Millennium by establishing a permanent clinic in this place, which can now be reached by Four-Wheel Drive vehicle in about two and a half hours from the hospital.

We thus complete an account of some developments of the clinics served by St. James' Hospital throughout the HSA of Mantšonyane.

It is difficult and challenging work to undertake, but the enthusiasm and hard work put into this vital work by the PHC team, second to none.

In the year 2000 it is earnestly hoped that a fresh donor for the whole Primary Health Care Programme will be found. The impact of this most worthwhile outreach is inestimable in terms of the long term care of the Basotho. They have benefited so much from having both curative and preventive care, brought to the area where they live, without having to face long and hazardous journeys to find medical and nursing aid. It has enabled them to lead much healthier lives.

Astounding progress has been made over the last 40 years. Those, who have made this wonderful work possible, are to be congratulated, as are the recipients of help. Without their co-operation and help, the implementation of Primary Health Care would not have been possible. Indeed it is probably true to say, that local people's involvement, has led to greater appreciation of the benefits received and ensured a considerable long term effect on health improvement.

CHAPTER 13 PAST, PRESENT and FUTURE

'God will remember how you have helped his people in the past and how you are still helping them.' (Heb. 6. 10. CEV)

PAST and PRESENT.

This account of the history of St. James' Hospital, Mantšonyane, has taken two years to complete, hopefully giving a realistic picture of a pioneer Christian medical project. It continues to serve the Basotho in the central mountainous region of one of Africa's poorest countries. The development of the project, which began in 1961, has been outlined from the earliest days to the present. When we arrived in what was virtually virgin territory from a medical viewpoint, we had little conception of how things would progress. Development has been made possible by the many and varied successors, who have been supported by churches and international organisations located all over the world - Australia, Canada, France, Germany, Eire, the Netherlands, RSA, and the United Kingdom and from Lesotho itself. Through their financial support and interest, they have helped in the accomplishments of one of the last mission hospitals to be established by the Church in the 20thC. Hopefully the gratitude and appreciation of the Basotho is reflected in these pages.

As in the West, the Church has been the pioneering influence in health and education, paving the way for governmental and secular agencies to continue. Even so, in a Third World country like Lesotho, there remains still a place for some ex-patriate workers, in a supportive role. In Lesotho, half the hospitals are still run by and substantially financed by the church, with additional government help from international organisations.

Although there are an increasing number of African doctors of a high calibre, few are willing to work for any length of time in an isolated place. In addition, they expect reasonable remuneration on a par with that of a government salary, particularly if they have a family to support. Many are drawn into private practice.

As first resident doctor at Mantšonyane, I was part of a team, which was responsible for introducing modern medical facilities on a regular basis to the local Basotho. It was necessary to learn a great deal about Sesotho beliefs and customs and to try to understand their underlying philosophy of life in order to help them, without riding rough shod over deeply held and often valuable traditional values. It was a reciprocal learning process. They had much to teach us and at the same time we had much to offer.

Forty years ago in this remote area, traditional beliefs and practices were not far below the surface whether patients were Christian or not. They were in the process of wisely blending the best of the old with the best of the new. This synthesis continues today. Even many urbanised Basotho, to a certain extent, retain traditional notions, some of which still have value. A parallel can be seen in the West, where traditional complementary therapies are being increasingly used in conjunction with orthodox medicine.

The traditional rural Basotho are still part of an extended family, but as more enter into modern urbanised society, this is breaking down. Just as in the West, they are beginning to experience the loneliness and isolation a more egocentric lifestyle brings. Another important difference is that traditional African religion covers all aspects of life, with no division between the sacred and the secular. This concept is mirrored in the life of the Church in Lesotho, for example ancestral veneration makes it easier to understand the Communion of Saints.

The role of traditional African healers has always been acknowledged and respected in the work at St. James' and in the PHC programmes. Courses, which have been organised for Traditional Healers, are not aimed at undermining their authority, but rather at making them appreciate that in some situations, hospital or clinic treatment is essential. Simultaneously doctors, nurses and ancillary staff learn of traditional remedies, some of which are beneficial. On the other hand, a factor which has to be emphasised, is that some are highly detrimental to health. The mutual understanding and exchange of knowledge has been to the patients benefit. Some types of mental illness do respond to traditional approaches. Certainly in my own experience the Church's Ministry of Healing has an important part to play.

MISSIONARIES of TODAY.

Today missionaries have a very different attitude to the stereotyped image of those in the past. Going to countries, like Lesotho, demands a flexible approach and willingness to learn. Many, myself included, would say that more was learnt about human life than ever was taught. Certainly living in a Third World country makes one aware of what really matters in life. A period overseas as a student quite often leads to them returning for a longer time before settling down to their chosen career. Mutual exchanges can be beneficial, but not always.

A most amusing scenario is related by David Fosbuary, a priest, who worked at Ha Chooko in 1970:

I arrived at a village in the evening after a day's trekking and slept the night there. In the morning some village ladies noticed me brushing my teeth and surmised that it was a purification ritual in preparation for celebrating Mass. So three of them asked at the store if they could order toothbrushes and toothpaste. The store keeper did not realise, when he ordered extra tubes of toothpaste, that it would be several years before they would be bought, as the ladies brushed their teeth only ten to twelve times a year when the peripatetic priest visited their village. At other times they cleaned them in the traditional ways they had learnt in childhood.

Much of this book may appear disjointed, but this reflects how life actually is, when things have to be dealt with as they occur. In Africa, one develops patience. Time is immaterial!

PAST ACHIEVEMENTS and DIFFICULTIES

Despite the multiple sources from which this book has been compiled there emerges a common objective, which is summed up in the word 'compassion'; (suffering with and helping each other). Among the different people, who served at Mantšonyane, there are remarkable similarities in comments and references to recurring problems; water supplies, staffing, finance or health matters. However as the hospital develops and circumstances change new problems arise, notably the increase in AIDS. Poverty is aggravated by increased unemployment as fewer men now find work in the mines of the RSA. In addition the influx of construction workers connected with the new dams at Katse and Mohale has brought some social and health problems for the local Basotho communities.

The story in this book has relevance for those who continue the work at present and in the future.

At times the work has been hampered by lack of continuity, though in recent years the helpful overlap of service by Dutch doctors has reduced the problem. Maybe it would be useful for future doctors, if a regularly updated journal could be kept at the hospital.

St. James' Hospital now serves approximately 64 000 Basotho (twice the number of 40 years ago), scattered throughout 80 square miles in the Maloti Mountains. It is one of the eight Church hospitals, which supplement the nine Government hospitals. The Mantšonyane HSA, one of the eighteen HSAs covering the whole country, is located in Thaba Moea and Hloahloeng, two of the poorest constituencies of Lesotho. Only 15% of the adult Basotho have paid employment and about 10% of Basotho households are able adequately to support themselves with food crops. 80% of the people own livestock, but as a result of overgrazing and inadequate fodder supplies, they are poor in quality. The majority of households live below the poverty line, particularly in remote areas.

Since St. James' Hospital opened in 1963, some needs have remained constant. Injuries are still the commonest cause for attendance, accounting for 20% of the outpatient workload. Of these, two thirds are the result of physical assault, often associated with alcohol abuse and fighting with sticks.

Gastro-intestinal infections represent a quarter of hospital admissions, explicable by the continued lack of sanitation and clean water supplies to many households, apart from in Lesobeng.. There has been an increase in the sexually transmitted diseases, now the second commonest reason for consultation. The emergence of Acquired Immune Deficiency Syndrome (AIDS) has become an increasing problem. Numbers have risen sharply from one HIV positive patient in 1991 to 115 in 1999 to 2000. Required hospital admission for AIDS related conditions, accounts for 10-11% of admissions and 10% of deaths in hospital. About one in three HIV positive patients will develop full- blown AIDS. The AIDS Prevention Programme at Mantšonyane is striving to educate local people about the need for protected sex, if a major epidemic is to be averted. In the year 2000, at Mantšonyane, it is likely that more than a hundred new HIV positive patients will be diagnosed, of whom a third will probably die. These patients, especially if malnourished, are susceptible to severe inter-current opportunistic infections, which can often be alleviated by enthusiastic treatment. In the country as a whole, deaths due to AIDS, it is anticipated, could exceed 1000 in the year 2000. Beds not utilised at present are therefore, likely to be occupied in the future by the ever increasing numbers of AIDS patients. At present 25 % of patients attending St. James' are now HIV positive, compared with 35 % in the country as a whole.

Chest infections are the next commonest problem and appear to be increasing. One in four hospital admissions are for TB as, sadly, the bacillus has become resistant to the drugs used. Chest infections in children remain a problem, often associated with malnutrition. Maternity admissions have fallen over recent years, to represent 6% of the total number. In part this is the result of better ante-natal care and training of Traditional Birth Attendants (TBAs.). Of those who do deliver in hospital, the number having Caesarean Sections has doubled. In all, 12 000 babies have been delivered since 1961! Heart and circulatory problems are more commonly seen and now, equal genito-urinary cases.

More than 25, 000 operations and about 30, 000 immunisations have been carried out since 1961. Major surgery is now performed more than once a week at St. James' Hospital and minor surgery, about twelve times a week at the hospital and clinics. Mainly this includes tooth extraction, suturing wounds and plastering fractures. The commonest causes of death are AIDS, TB. and pneumonia. Measles no longer seems to be a killer.

The full impact of the tremendous growth and development of St. James' Hospital and its work was brought home to me and my wife, when we were privileged to revisit Lesotho in April 1999. We were part of a group of 15 supporters of the Lesotho Diocesan Association, based in the UK. As the first and longest serving doctor at Mantšonyane, it was a great and partially unexpected joy to be able to see firsthand all that had been accomplished since I arrived with the original team, 38 years before. At that stage the Mountain Road had only recently reached Manšonyane and it literally ended at the trading store on the edge of the small village of Ha Toka, half a mile from the site of the future hospital. Now the Mountain Road goes right through to the Drakensberg Mountains via Thaba Tseka and Mokhotlong and thus into Natal. We were intrigued to read in the visitors' brochure that Mantšonyane was referred to as a 'town'!. There certainly had been a transformation. It now has two trading stores, selling a wide range of food and household goods including furniture! A multitude of small vendors are located round the village and along the road. Perhaps the most impressive development is the recently opened Post Office, a palatial building by anyone's standard.

A clear sign directed our Mosotho driver around the corner to 'St. James' Hospital, Anglican Church of Lesotho'. As we turned into the entrance , we saw a veritable cluster of buildings enveloped by many well established trees. Originally the whole area was a bare plateau. We were delighted to see that some of the 3000 trees, which we had planted, had survived to maturity. The front of the hospital was easily identified by the huge cross over the main entrance. However, so much building had taken place, that it took two days to discover all the extensions and additions.

On our arrival, Dr. Simone Jaarsma, the Medical Superintendent, was busy in the operating theatre performing a Caesarean Section for a lady, who had ruptured her uterus. We were first shown into the board -room in the Administration Block where we ate our buffet lunch with the LDA. Around the giant satellite television, were gathered some of the off duty staff keenly watching international football coverage. They seemed to be far more knowledgeable about Manchester United than many of us! After lunch we were welcomed by Dr. Simone, who showed us around the main buildings. The outpatient department had much improved facilities for minor surgery. A small white rondavel chapel, with the old natural stone altar and aumbry from the original chapel, were integrated into the hospital building. The operating theatre had been updated as well as the delivery suite. A new midwifery ward, a premature baby unit, equipped with incubators and proper waiting facilities for pregnant mothers were further additions, together with 'Ultra sound'. The old laundry now serves as a sunny male ward, with isolation facilities for AIDS patients. In the new laundry, an industrial sized washing machine copes speedily and hygienically with hospital linen. The twenty-bedded female ward, built in 1965, is still in full use. In all the total number of beds is 60 compared with 35 thirty years ago.

There are many other new buildings, but perhaps one of the most significant is the headquarters of the PHC. It serves as the co-ordinating centre for all the outstation clinics and is also used by the social services. It also offers greater privacy for counselling HIV patients.

The whole hospital complex now has a 24 hours a day electricity supply and a reliable water supply. Both are from local sources. The boundaries of the hospital compound have been extended considerably to allow for a larger and much improved airstrip, which gives easier access for the LFDS, to Maseru and some of the clinics.

Staff members have increased from 20 in 1968 to 50 in 1999 at the hospital itself. These include three doctors, a matron assisted by five sisters, a registered nurse and ten nursing assistants plus 30 ancillary staff. These is a water engineer from Nepal, a social worker, pharmaceutical and some laboratory technicians, as well as the maintenance team and Rob van Akker, Simone's husband, who acts as technical advisor for the hospital and clinics. Each fulfils a vital role in the smooth running of the hospital. In addition, the District Public Health Team are now based in the hospital compound. St James' Hospital is well run and provides excellent medical care, with Dr. Simone as Medical Superintendent. Since she had now become responsible for the PHC, the new doctor, Dr. Deji Falodu from Nigeria, who had recently joined the medical staff, would be in charge of hospital care. Over the last 20 years, the number of outpatients attending the hospital and clinics has doubled. Since 1961, the cumulative total is nearing three quarters of a million. Inpatients total about 30 000 since 1963. Interestingly the inpatient numbers have been decreasing. There are two probable explanations for this. Firstly, it is the result of more effective preventive health care, carried out by the PHC in the clinics, and secondly it is a question of finance. Some patients are unable to pay the fees. However, there is a 'poor fund' financed by the Glovers and Skinners Corporation of Glasgow, Scotland, to be used for the very poor needing urgent treatment.

THE CHRISTIAN CONTEXT.

The original stimulus for the work of St James' Hospital came from the Anglican Church through the substantial efforts of the Society for the Propagation of the Gospel. The hospital remains the responsibility of the Anglican Church of Lesotho. However its running costs are still substantially met from the sustained support of individual parishes through the Project Scheme of USPG. The Diocese of Lesotho is financially poor, but it offers spiritual care and support to the hospital, its staff and patients.

At Mantšonyane, the new church, rectory and school have been built next to the hospital and the rector takes an active part on the hospital board and as chaplain to the hospital. Father Aubrey Ntho, however, expressed his anxiety at having to be away for six weeks at a time visiting outstations. There is a need for continuous pastoral care for the staff and the patients. Therefore, hopefully more trained lay Basotho will be a priority for the new Bishop of Lesotho, Joseph Tsubella.

In a recent newsletter, he had this to say:

I was impressed by the work the staff is doing and I think the hospital is playing a very important role in the mountains. In an area like this the hospital is 'like a source of water to supply life in the desert'. And I think the hospital needs a lot of support. People would have died if there would not have been a hospital. And thank God that more clinics have sprung up to bring the services even closer to the people. Because of the mountains transport is always difficult and costly and it is good to have clinics nearby. The community should be proud of the hospital.

The role of the staff is very important, we shouldn't forget how much they sacrifice. It could have been easy for them to find work elsewhere

and earn better salaries. Good staff is even more important than buildings and equipment, they are the ones who do the real work. In that way the staff are doing what Jesus told us: 'I have come that you may have life and have it in abundance'. It is important to save the lives of the people first and worry about the money later. Still people do not come to the hospital because of personal financial problems. It is good that the hospital has some facilities to take care of people who have no money at all but who really need help.

At the moment there are not many Anglicans in key positions in the hospital. It would good if there were more Anglicans actively involved in the hospital. Anglicans should also be represented in health services if possible. The Anglicans should realise that lives are at risk without a hospital and that they have an important role to play. Of course a hospital needs professional staff and therefore qualifications are the most important aspect.

The work as it is done now in St. James' is as Jesus would have done it. It is like a ministry. Taking care of the people is what Jesus is expecting of people. The staff is doing a great job. And the hospital needs support from everybody who also thinks that this work is important.

The return of the Sisters of the Holy Name to the hospital would be very welcome for improving pastoral care, if this were possible.

Compared with the very early days, the Eucharist today forms a marked contrast with that of the first one in March 1962, when Fr. Donald Hiscock celebrated in the workshop-cum-stable with the carpenter's bench serving as an altar, and the congregation kneeling on the concrete floor. Thirty-seven years later, it was a great joy to preach a Sesotho sermon in the new church. The text chosen was, 'I lift my eyes to the mountains. From where will my help come? My help will come from the Lord who made both heaven and earth' (Psalm 121). When I reminded them of the early days, our old friends, who were among the congregation, were moved when I spoke of the old name of the hospital site, 'khaula', a place of compassion. Truly it had become a place of compassion, serving the people of the Maloti. Only through the efforts of people throughout the world and those who had worked at St. James' had this been possible. I said, 'Like Morena Chooko, we should lift up our eyes to the Lord, who made the Maloti Mountains. Truly God will continue to provide for his works of compassion, right in this part of his Kingdom. Today we bring greetings to you all from Christians of England. Together we share the joy of the resurrection of our Lord Jesus Christ and his new life'.

We closed with the prayer of St. James' Hospital, of which an English translation is given at the end of this chapter. At the sharing of the Peace, I was moved to tears of joy!

URGENT NEEDS.

Having outlined the general opportunities for service and the needs of pastoral care, it is necessary to turn to serious concerns which could jeopardise the continuation of work at St. James'. Crises have occurred in the past and miraculously have been overcome. As the present Medical Superintendent would verify there are three major problems:

1. THE CONTINUATION OF THE PHC PROGRAMME

Until a year ago, the EZE of Germany sponsored this highly effective and much valued work. With the cessation of this support, hospital funds now have to be used to maintain the clinics and health centres.

In her letter dated 29th February 2000, Dr. Jaarsma said:

We are still looking for a donor for the PHC Programme. Christian Aid (London) may be interested and I hope to meet a representative from Christian Aid soon. If we do not find a PHC sponsor this year I am afraid that we may have to cease all our PHC activities. The transport component especially consumes a lot of money. The hospital has carried the burden for the past year or more and the deficit is increasing!'

Whether or not Christian Aid takes over support of the PHC, it may well be that more than one sponsor will be required to maintain it effectively in the long term. It is good to know that USPG have agreed to sponsor half the running costs of the PHC.

2. FUTURE MEDICAL STAFFING OF THE HOSPITAL.

In her recent letter Dr. Jaarsma imparts some sad news:

I will not be replaced by another Dutch doctor when my contract ends in February 2001. Policies in the Netherlands have changed and the DOG will no longer send a Dutch doctor if someone can be found locally. I am trying through the Diocese of Lesotho to find a replacement for me, who may be an Anglican missionary doctor.

This is a serious blow to the hospital, which for the last 20 years has relied on a continual succession of excellent Dutch doctors. One can appreciate the decision of the DOG in the Netherlands, who consider that local African doctors should be employed in preference to expatriate ones. However to date, no Mosotho doctor has been willing to work there and those African doctors, who have given excellent service, have not stayed for any length of time. In part, the explanation may lie in the isolation of Mantšonyane. Dr Jaarsma has suggested the possibility of an Anglican Mission doctor. The plain fact is that Anglican doctors have never been offered a realistic salary, unlike the Dutch doctors whose payment by their Government has been on a par with salaries in the Netherlands. Gone are the days of heroic sacrifice in terms of finance. Doctors working overseas are already making sacrifice in terms of an interrupted professional career and they are often working in a lonely environment. A fair salary is essential to possible future recruitment. Lesotho is a British Commonwealth country and may be the Ministry of Overseas Development could be approached regarding sponsorship for future hospital doctors. Alternatively help may come from world-wide organisations or other countries.

Another point to bear in mind is that the appointment of a competent administrator would relieve pressure on the doctors' workload and provide continuity. Serious efforts should be made to recruit such a person for several year periods- possibly an experienced person who has taken early retirement.

3. FINANCIAL SUPPORT.

Christian hospitals make a significant contribution towards the health of the Kingdom of Lesotho. However they are unable to pay salaries equivalent to those of the Government hospitals. In order to attract staff, particularly nurses and maintenance staff of the right calibre, salaries need to be supplemented. Negotiations with the Government have been going on for years, with no satisfactory conclusion. Were financial support to materialise, it would be possible to close the disparity in fees between Government and Christian hospitals. At present the Christian hospitals, which tend to be in the remoter areas of the country, are forced to charge higher amounts. This often means that local Basotho are unable to make full use of the available facilities.

In the past, parish support through USPG has provided an important source of income, but at present this represents only about 50% of the running costs of the hospital. Increased support would be greatly appreciated through USPG as well as through the LDA and private donors.

Direct links with overseas dioceses, for example, the Durham-Lesotho Link, are likely to be increasingly important, not only for particular projects which generate keen interest, but also for general maintenance costs, which are likely to rise.

Help is urgently needed for St. James' to continue its vital work.

Please remember St. James' Hospital in your thoughts and prayers. You may like to use the following prayer, which is based on the Prayer of St. James' Hospital:

'O God, you have revealed your compassion in the life and passion of your dear Son; continue your compassion through the work of St. James' Hospital and all who serve there; that suffering with Christ, and caring for those who suffer in body, mind and spirit, they may continue to heal in your name and for your sake.

Through Jesus Christ our Lord. Amen'

THE END.

SESOTHO- ENGLISH VOCABULARY.

Bakhachane- pregnant women.
Basotho- people of Lesotho.
Batsoetse- newly delivered mothers.
Bukana- little book for persona patient records.
Ente- injection.
Ha- place of.
Joala- Sesotho beer.
Kereke ea Chache- Anglican Church.
`*Me*- mother.
`*Missa*- Mass.
Mokete- feast.
Mokakalane- Spanish influenza epidemic of 1918.
Morena- chief.
Mosotho- singular of Basotho.
Ngaka- doctor.
Ntate- father
Ntoa ea Lithunya- Gun War of 1880.
Pitso- meeting.
Sepetlele- hospital.
Sesotho- language and customs of the Basotho.

USEFUL ADDRESSES:

The Bishop of Lesotho,
P.O. Box 87, Maseru 100, Lesotho, Southern Africa

Lesotho Diocesan Association,
86, King's Road, Oakham, Rutland, LE15 6 PD UK..

Durham- Lesotho Link,
Diocesan Office, Auckland Castle, Bishop Auckland,
Co. Durham, DL14 7Q.J. UK

St. James' Hospital,
P.O. Box 3, Mantšonyane150, Lesotho, Southern Africa

The United Society for the Propagation of the Gospel,
157, Waterloo Road, London, SE1 8XA UK

Other titles published by Authors Online Ltd.

FICTION

By Peter Townsend

The Forties Man - ISBN 0-7552-0008-X - £9.95
Trevor must save Saltfleet from an unexploded bomb, with only a stuffed dog, some mismatched allies and the spirit of the Blitz to help him.

The Jet Stone – ISBN 0-7552-0003-9 - £11.95
Following the disappearance of two women in Whitby in the 1880s there is a frantic attempt to find them by two feuding cousins before it is too late.

The Flying Star – ISBN 0-7552-0005-5 - £8.95
Volunteers running a miniature railway are faced with a stark choice of having to commit a murder, or instead see their railway destined for the scrapheap.

By Wendy Anne Lake

Cinder Path – ISBN 0-7552-0017-9 - £8.95
Poignant family saga set in the heart of Lancashire. A sexually steamy story of jealousy, rejection, betrayal and loss. Will Vicky ever find the love she yearns for with Jim.

Inspired Urges – ISBN 0-7552-0019-5 - £12.95
A scintillating saga of rags to riches set on both sides of the Atlantic. Filled with deep sexual prowess and a dangerous ambition.

Sensual Rhythm of Perfect Melody – ISBN 0-7552-0010-1 - £11.95
Melody finds herself beautifully seduced by a tall stranger. In the midst of lust, she is asked what Mel is short for and thoughtlessly gasps out Melody. The consequences are more than far reaching as she descends into a life of an erotic dancer and sex object.

Labyrinth of Desire – ISBN 0-7552-0013-6 - £9.95
The sensual Evie Warrender trains alongside her idol, the handsome, eminent barrister, Bruce Manning. She is stunned one evening, when out of the blue, he leads her into the realms of exotic passion and an excitement she never knew existed

---

By Nick Wastnage

The Electronic Conspirator - ISBN 0-7552-0007-1 - £11.95
The most unlikely man pulls off the perfect electronic scam. He sets up five innocent, but desperate people, kills himself and escapes with the money: leaving behind a scorned ex-lover and a bitter ex-wife. His tranquillity is short-lived

---

By Tony Stowell

A Little Learning – ISBN 0-7552-0006-3 - £11.95
A work of fiction set in a secondary school that has some deadly accurate messages about the state of education today. A 'must' for all teachers and parents!

The Woolsack Conspiracy – ISBN 0-7552-0011-X - £11.95
A young man has his values turned upside down in this tense thriller, where terrorism meets rural tradition, and where romance and passion are never far from the surface.

By Desmond Tarrant

Power & Beauty – ISBN 0-7552-0015-2 - £12.95
Told with colour and humour, this outstanding novel is based on the truth. It ranges from RAF Bomber Command over Germany in 1944/45 and the heady days of the British Raj in India to international finance and romance - a real pleasure to read.

The Firebrand – ISBN 0-7552-0014-4 - £11.95
This major novel offers first class entertainment and craftsmanship with the latest understanding of what life is all about. It is a real page-turner, essential, vital reading today.

By Alan Taylor

One Day As A Tiger – ISBN 0-7552-0020-9 - £11.95
The last two turbulent decades of the British Raj in India is the exciting setting for an unusual saga of romance and colour imaginatively conceived by an author who lived there at the time.

By Sonia Y Lasser

The Deadly Conference – ISBN 0-7552-0021-7 - £9.95

Top, international scientists agree to gather at a conference eager to present their solutions for cheap and clean energy. Racing against time, the scientists are working around the clock to prove the feasibility of the suggested idea stolen from the big, secret computer program. Strange and bizarre things happen on the way to the conference, scheduled in a resort town in Northern Italy. But who is trying to stop them from achieving their goal?

By Simon Kalik

Blissful Assassination – ISBN 0-7552-0018-7 - £11.95

A thriller that will shock you with its goriness and arouse you with its sexual adventures

By Peter Hughes

Closing Time – ISBN 0-7552-0024-1 - £8.95

A compelling lightheartedness tumbles the reader through the sticky pages of 'Closing Time': Bad behaviour in bedsit land, bar-room philosophy and bodily functions are but some of the juicy centres of this delicious story-telling.

By Susan Shaw

Eleanor – ISBN 0-7552-0026-8 - £11.95

A novel of strong emotional turmoil regarding a woman's strife trying to overcome conventions so as to be equal to the men in her life, after the First World War.

NON-FICTION

By Evelyn Stewart

Totally Discombobulated –ISBN 0-7552-0012-8 - £14.95
A true, and sometimes tragic, family drama covering a period from 1940 through 1982. The story vividly follows the life of our author as she courageously walks through a seemingly unending cessation of spousal abuse, murder, incest and a legacy of turmoil.

By Annette Willoughby

Innocent in Africa - ISBN 0-7552-0009-8 - £14.95
An amusing and poignant story of a teacher from South London who, on an overnight impulse, joins her partner in The Mountain Kingdom of Lesotho.

By Keats Babel

Ant Musings – ISBN 0-7552-0022-5 - £12.95
In 1980s London, Bandit Matthews was a rebellious youngster with strong opinions and a passion for Ant Music. Twenty years later, nothing much had changed…

By Wendy Anne Lake

You've Been Wonderful To Your Father - ISBN 0-7552-0004-7 - £11.95
A heartrending, yet uplifting story of a stroke victim and the tender love of his family.

By Simon Lee

Spiritual Energy 0-7552-0023-3 - £11.95
An 'anti-materialistic, 21st Century Spiritual Metaphysics' which submits that The Mind and The Spirit are Real and Exist in their own right – they are not just 'froth made out of chemicals'! This book provides instead a complete analysis of both the component qualities, and the structure, of Spiritual Energy.

To order a copy of any of the above please fill out this form and post it to.
Authors OnLine Ltd
15-17 Maidenhead Street
Hertford SG14 1DW
England

theeditor@authorsonline.co.uk

Author	Title	ISBN	Price
		Total	
		P&P @ £1.95 per Book	
		Total Due	

Address for Delivery

_____

_____

_____

Post Code_____

Cheque enclosed £_____

www.authorsonline.co.uk